Atlas of H
on C

Atlas of Human Anatomy on CT Imaging

(Brig) Hariqbal Singh MD DMRD
Professor and Head
Department of Radiology
Shrimati Kashibai Navale Medical College
Pune, Maharashtra (India)

Anubhav Khandelwal DNB
Senior Resident
Shrimati Kashibai Navale Medical College
Pune, Maharashtra (India)

Sushil Kachewar MD DNB
Assistant Professor
Shrimati Kashibai Navale Medical College
Pune, Maharashtra (India)

JAYPEE BROTHERS MEDICAL PUBLISHERS (P) LTD

New Delhi • St Louis (USA) • Panama City (Panama) • London (UK) • Ahmedabad
Bengaluru • Chennai • Hyderabad • Kolkata • Kochi • Lucknow • Mumbai • Nagpur

Published by
Jitendar P Vij
Jaypee Brothers Medical Publishers (P) Ltd

Corporate Office
4838/24 Ansari Road, Daryaganj, New Delhi - 110002, India,
Phone: +91-11-43574357, Fax: +91-11-43574314

Registered Office
B-3 EMCA House, 23/23B Ansari Road, Daryaganj, New Delhi - 110 002, India
Phones: +91-11-23272143, +91-11-23272703, +91-11-23282021
+91-11-23245672, Rel: +91-11-32558559, Fax: +91-11-23276490, +91-11-23245683
e-mail: jaypee@jaypeebrothers.com, Website: www.jaypeebrothers.com

Offices in India
- Ahmedabad, Phone: Rel: +91-79-32988717
  e-mail: ahmedabad@jaypeebrothers.com
- Bengaluru, Phone: Rel: +91-80-32714073
  e-mail: bangalore@jaypeebrothers.com
- Chennai, Phone: Rel: +91-44-32972089
  e-mail: chennai@jaypeebrothers.com
- Hyderabad, Phone: Rel:+91-40-32940929
  e-mail: hyderabad@jaypeebrothers.com
- Kochi, Phone: +91-484-2395740, e-mail: kochi@jaypeebrothers.com
- Kolkata, Phone: +91-33-22276415, e-mail: kolkata@jaypeebrothers.com
- Lucknow, Phone: +91-522-3040554, e-mail: lucknow@jaypeebrothers.com
- Mumbai, Phone: Rel: +91-22-32926896
  e-mail: mumbai@jaypeebrothers.com
- Nagpur, Phone: Rel: +91-712-3245220
  e-mail: nagpur@jaypeebrothers.com

Overseas Offices
- North America Office, USA, Ph: 001-636-6279734
  e-mail: jaypee@jaypeebrothers.com, anjulav@jaypeebrothers.com
- Central America Office, Panama City, Panama, Ph: 001-507-317-0160
  e-mail: cservice@jphmedical.com, Website: www.jphmedical.com
- Europe Office, UK, Ph: +44 (0) 2031708910, e-mail: dholman@jpmedical.biz

Atlas of Human Anatomy on CT Imaging

This book has been published in good faith that the material provided by authors is original. Every effort is made to ensure accuracy of material, but the publisher, printer and authors will not be held responsible for any inadvertent error(s). In case of any dispute, all legal matters are to be settled under Delhi jurisdiction only.

First Edition: 2010
ISBN 978-81-8448-940-8
Typeset at JPBMP typesetting unit
Printed at Replika Press Pvt. Ltd.

This book is dedicated to our inspiring and loving parents
Harnam Singh and *Kishan Kaur*
Harish and *Padma Khandelwal*
Ghanshyam and *Vidya Kachewar*

"University is a nursery of scientific research and mental education". "Pride in one's profession is demanded, but not professional conceit, snobbery or academic arrogance, all of which grow from false egoism."

From the inaugural address of Wilhelm Conrad Roentgen, on being appointed by the University of Würzburg as the Director of Physical Institute in 1894, a year before his discovery of X-rays.

PREFACE

Human anatomy has not changed but the advances in imaging modalities have changed our perception of structural and functional details. This book is loaded with meticulously labeled cross-sectional CT scan images of normal human anatomy which is a prerequisite for identifying the pathology. With each image the topogram shows the level of the section which enhances the understanding of anatomy. Undergraduate as well as postgraduate medical students will find this book extremely useful.

(Brig) Hariqbal Singh
Anubhav Khandelwal
Sushil Kachewar

ACKNOWLEDGMENTS

We thank Prof MN Navale, Founder President, Sinhgad Technical Educational Society and Dr Arvind V Bhore, Dean, Smt Kashibai Navale Medical College for their kind permission in this endeavor.

Any accomplishment requires the effort of many people and this work is no different. We express our gratitude to the entire Staff of Imaging Department of this institution.

We would like to extend our thanks to faculty members, Dr Anand Kamat, Prashant Naik, Abhijit Pawar, Sushant Bhadane, Santosh Konde, Amol Sasane, Rajlaxmi Sharma, Sheetal Dhote, Mrunalini Shah, Amol Nade and Rahul Tupe who have helped in compiling the images.

We thank Dr Smita Khandelwal for her generous contribution of CT angiography images.

Our special thanks to the CT Scan Technicians Mr More Rahul, Demello Thomas, Musmade Bala, Raghvendra and Mrs Manjusha Chikale nursing sister and receptionist of the CT unit for their untiring help in retrieving the data.

We thank our Artist cum Photographer Mr Sanjay Raut for developing on certain images and Mrs Snehal Nikalje for her clerical help.

We are grateful to God and mankind who have allowed us to have this wonderful experience.

CONTENTS

INTRODUCTION

CT is a diagnostic imaging procedure to obtain cross-sectional images of the body by use of X-rays. CT overcomes the limitation of plain radiography where three dimensional structures are shown in two dimensions only. Since its introduction in the 1970s; it has become recognized as a valuable medical tool not only for the diagnosing abnormality but also for planning, guiding and monitoring the appropriate therapy.

In a CT scan, different angular X-ray projections are processed with the help of a computer to provide a matrix of picture elements (pixels). All of the tissues contained within the pixel attenuate the X-ray projections and result in a mean attenuation value for that pixel. This value is compared with the attenuation value of water and is displayed on a scale (Hounsfield Scale). Water is allotted attenuation value of zero Hounsfield units (0 HU). Air is – 800 to – 1000 HU; fat is approximately – 80 to – 100 HU; soft tissues are in the range + 20 to + 70 HU and bone is usually greater than + 350 HU. The scale is 2000 HU wide.

Modern multislice helical CT scanners obtain images in sub-second and hence imaging of the whole body can take as little as a single breath hold of 20-30 seconds. This fast scan times allow dynamic imaging of arteries and veins.

Digital images are stored in an electronic storage record known as PACS (Picture archiving and communication system), that enables the interrogation and visualization of images via an electronic network at any desired place.

Most CT scans are performed with the patient in supine position and images are obtained in axial plain. Images can also be taken at upto 20-25 degrees of gantry angulation, which is valuable for spine imaging. Direct coronal images with neck in extended position are obtained for cranial, PNS and maxillofacial pathologies.

For CT examinations intravenous iodine containing contrast medium is required to show differential enhancement of normal and pathological tissues and to demonstrate the arteries and veins. Bowel opacification is provided by means of oral water soluble contrast medium in CT abdomen and pelvis. Oral contrast is given four hours prior to the examination to show the colon, followed by further oral intake at around zero to sixty minutes prior to the scan, for outlining upper GIT. Direct insertion of rectal contrast and air with Higginson's syringe demonstrates the distal large bowel better.

Usage of CT exposes a patient to significant radiation; hence benefit versus risk analysis is a must prior to submitting a patient for CT scan.

Plate 1

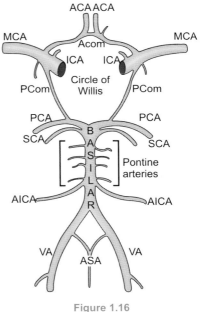

ACA–Anterior cerebral artery;
ACom–Anterior communicating
   artery;
MCA–Middle cerebral artery;
ICA–Internal carotid artery;
PCom–Posterior
   communicating artery;
PCA–Posterior cerebral artery;
SCA–Superior cerebellar artery;
BASILAR–Basilar artery;
AICA–Anterior inferior cerebellar
   artery;
VA–Vertebral artery;
ASA–Anterior spinal artery.

Figure 1.16

Plate 2

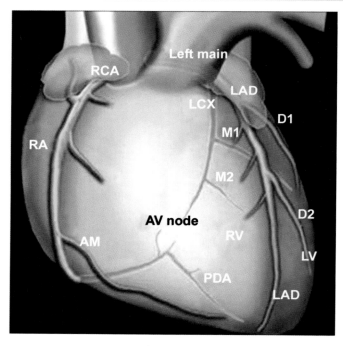

Figure 7.1

Plate 3

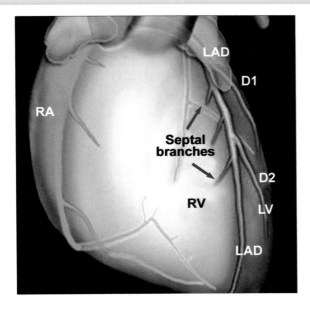

Figure 7.2

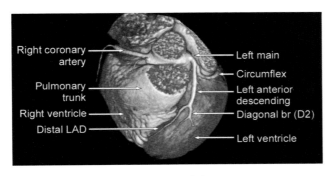

Figure 7.3: Axial plane

Plate 4

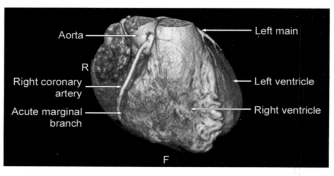

Figure 7.4: Coronal plane

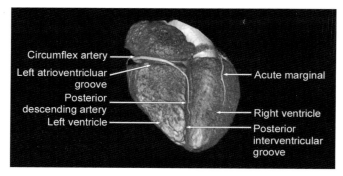

Figure 7.5: Posterior coronal plane

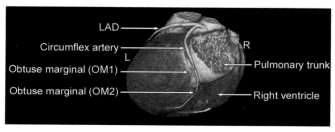

Figure 7.6: Posterior oblique coronal plane

Plate 5

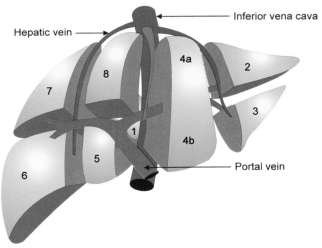

Figure 8.1

1 Brain

Brain is enclosed in the cranium which includes all the bones that make the skeleton of head and are joined to each other with help of joints known as sutures. Inner part of skull base is divided into anterior, middle and posterior cranial fossae.

Skull base has multiple foramen through which various nerves and vessels pass.

Foramen Rotandum situated in greater wing of sphenoid connects middle cranial fossa and pterygopalatine fossa. Maxillary division of trigeminal nerve, artery of foramen Rotandum and an emissary vein pass through it.

Foramen Lacerum is located at lower aspect of medial pterygoid plate. Nerve to pterygoid canal and meningeal branch of ascending pharyngeal artery pass through it.

Foramen Spinosum is situated in greater wing of sphenoid posterolateral to foramen ovale. Middle meningeal artery and vein and lesser superficial petrosal nerve and meningeal branch of mandibular nerve pass through it.

Foramen Ovale connects infratemporal fossa and middle cranial fossa. Mandibular division of trigeminal nerve, lesser petrosal nerve, accessory meningeal artery and emissary vein pass through it.

Foramen Magnum is located in the occipital bone. It contains medulla oblongata, spinal accessory nerve, vertebral artery and spinal arteries.

Jugular foramen is located at posterior end of petro-occipital suture. Inferior petrosal sinus, meningeal branches of pharyngeal artery and occipital artery pass through its anterior part. IXth, Xth and XIth cranial nerves pass through its intermediate part. Internal jugular vein is located in its posterior most part.

Orbitomeatal line is an imaginary line running from external auditory meatus to superior wall of orbit. Sections of CT scan of brain are taken parallel to this line.

Embryologically brain develops from neural plate which arises from the ectoderm on dorsal aspect of embryo at around 4-5 weeks of intrauterine life. Maximum growth occurs in the second trimester. Pattern of myelination extends caudocranially and posteroanteriorly.

Anatomically brain is divided into forebrain (Prosencephalon), midbrain (Mesencephalon) and hindbrain (Rhombencephalon).

Forebrain (Prosencephalon) consists of:

a. Cererbrum (Telencephalon) includes cerebral hemispheres, caudate nucleus and putamen.
b. Diencephalon includes epithalamus (pineal gland), thalamus, hypothalamus and globus pallidus.

Parts of midbrain (Mesencephalon) consist of corpora quadri-gemina, tectum, cerebral peduncles and suprapontine portion.

Hindbrain (Rhombencephalon) consists of:

a. Metencephalon which includes cerebellar hemispheres and the vermis.
b. Myelencephalon made of pons and medulla oblongata.

Brainstem is composed of Mesencephalon and Myelence-phalon. Cranial nerve nuclei are located in the brainstem.

The cross-section of head shows:

1. Scalp which has following five layers from outside inwards: skin, subcutaneous fibro-adipose layer, galea aponeurotica, subgaleal areolar tissue layer and pericranium.
2. Calvarium or skull table which includes inner and outer tables of bones. Outer table is made of strong compact bone. Inner table has thin brittle compact bone. Diplopic space between these two skull tables is made of trabecular bone and is filled by red marrow.

3. Meninges of the brain include the outer pachymeninges (dura mater) and inner leptomeninges (arachnoid and pia mater).

Subperiosteal space is between calvarium and periosteum of outer skull table. Bleeding here leads to cephalohematoma.

Epidural or extradural space is between periosteum of inner skull table and calvarium.

Subdural space is within inner layer of dura and arachnoid mater. Subarachnoid space exists between arachnoid and pia mater. Subpial space is the perivascular Virchow-Robin space that exists in brain.

Cerebrospinal fluid fills the entire ventricular system, sulci and cisterns. There is 150 ml of total CSF in an adult. It is produced at the rate of 0.4 ml/min by choroid plexuses in the lateral ventricles. The flow is as follows:

From lateral ventricles it enters the third ventricle via foramen of Monro. From third ventricle it goes through aqueduct of Sylvius and enters the fourth ventricle. Foramen of Luschka and foramen of Magendie are the outlets of CSF from fourth ventricle to various sulci and cisterns surrounding brain. From these sulci and cisterns CSF is absorbed in the venous system through arachnoid villae. Small amount also continues into the CSF filled spinal canal located at center of spinal cord.

Each part of brain has an outer gray matter (collection of nerve cells) and an inner white matter (nerve fibers and tracts).

Basal ganglia is a group of neurons lying deep within the cortex. Basal ganglia consists of Claustrum, Corpus striatum [Caudate + Lentiform nucleus (putamen and globus pallidus)] and Amygdaloid body.

Pituitary gland is located in the pituitary fossa of sphenoid bone, the roof of which is formed by diaphragma sellae. Pituitary gland has an anterior lobe, pars intermedia and a posterior lobe.

Brain is supplied by carotid and vertebral arteries. Common carotid artery divided into the internal carotid and external carotid branches. Internal carotid supplies the brain. It has cervical, petrous, cavernous and supraclinoid segments. Supraclinoid segment gives rise to anterior and middle cerebral arteries. Posterior cerebral artery arises from basilar artery which is formed after fusion of vertebral arteries.

The arterial anastomoses of the brain is called as the Circle of Willis which is contributed to by the anterior, middle and posterior cerebral arteries to supply blood to entire brain.

Cerebellum is supplied by anterior and posterior inferior cerebellar arteries and superior cerebellar arteries which arise from vertebro-basilar arteries which originates from subclavian artery or directly from aorta.

Various veins collect the blood from brain and drain into venous sinuses which drain into the internal jugular vein.

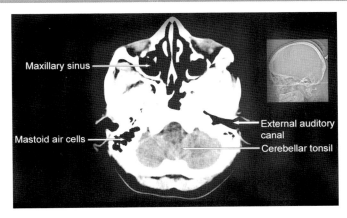

Figure 1.1: Axial CT section of brain

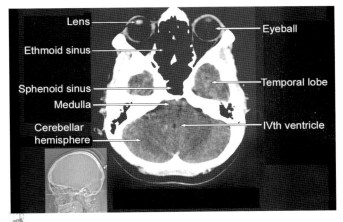

Figure 1.2: Axial CT section of brain

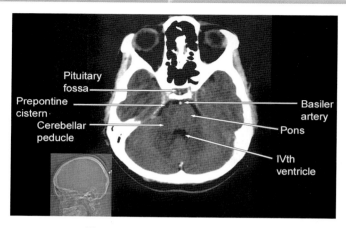

Figure 1.3: Axial CT section of brain

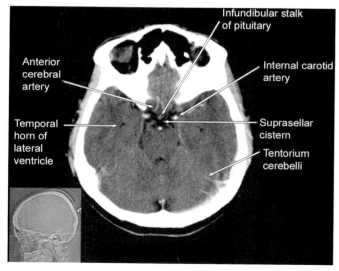

Figure 1.4: Axial CT section of brain

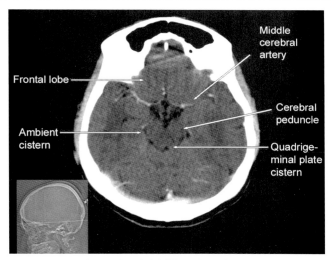

Figure 1.5: Axial CT section of brain

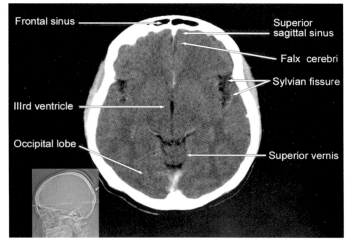

Axial CT section of brain

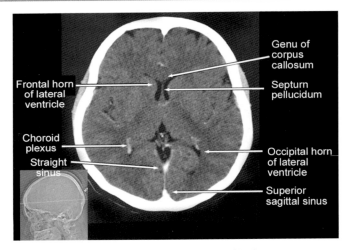

Figure 1.7: Axial CT section of brain

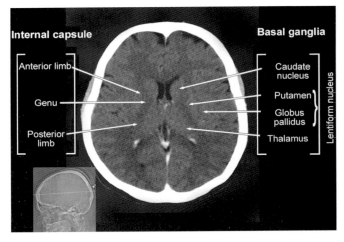

Figure 1.8: Axial CT section of brain

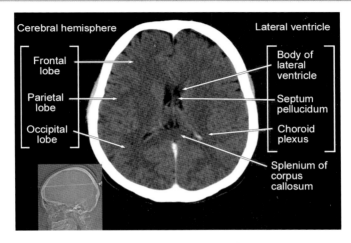

Figure 1.9: Axial CT section of brain

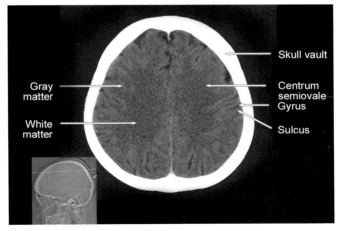

Figure 1.10: Axial CT section of brain

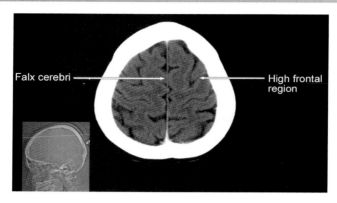

Figure 1.11: Axial CT section of brain

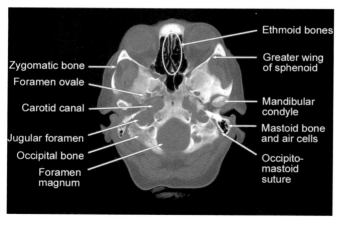

Figure 1.12: Axial CT section of brain in bone window

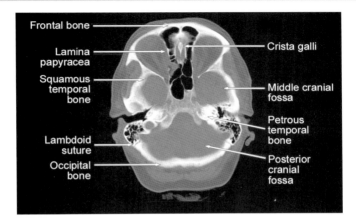

Figure 1.13: Axial CT section of head in bone window

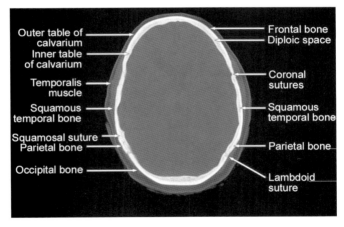

Figure 1.14: Axial CT section of head in bone window

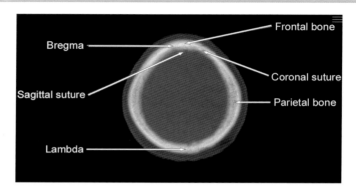

Figure 1.15: Axial CT section of head in bone window

ACA–Anterior cerebral artery;
ACom–Anterior communicating
    artery;
MCA–Middle cerebral artery;
ICA–Internal carotid artery;
PCom–Posterior
    communicating artery;
PCA–Posterior cerebral artery;
SCA–Superior cerebellar artery;
BASILAR–Basilar artery;
AICA–Anterior inferior cerebellar
    artery;
VA–Vertebral artery;
ASA–Anterior spinal artery.

Figure 1.16: (For color version see Plate 1)

ORBIT

Orbit is a pyramid shaped cavity. Roof of orbit is formed by orbital plate of the frontal bone. Medial wall is the thinnest and is formed by a small portion of the frontal process of maxilla, the lacrimal bone, the ethmoid bone and the body of sphenoid. Floor is made by the orbital part of maxillary bone. Lateral orbital wall is the thickest and is formed by orbital surface of the greater wing of sphenoid. Eyeball is the main structure of the anterior orbit; it is divided into small anterior chamber and larger posterior chamber (vitreous), by the lens. Optic nerve along with ophthalmic artery passes posteriorly into the middle cranial fossa through the optic canal. Superior orbital fissure is present between the greater and lesser wings of sphenoid. Oculomotor, Trochlear and Abducent nerves (III, IV and VI cranial nerves), lacrimal, frontal and nasal branches of the trigeminal nerve, ophthalmic veins and anterior connections between the middle meningeal and ophthlamic artery passes through the superior orbital fissure. Inferior orbital fissure lies between the lateral and inferior orbital walls and emissary veins pass through it.

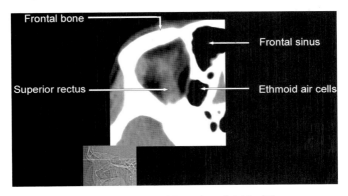

Figure 1.17: Axial CT section of right orbit

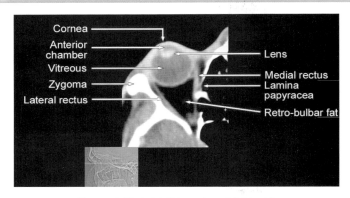

Figure 1.18: Axial CT section of right orbit

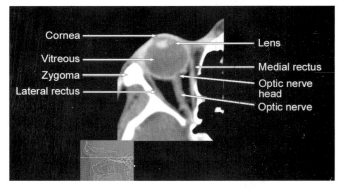

Figure 1.19: Axial CT section of right orbit

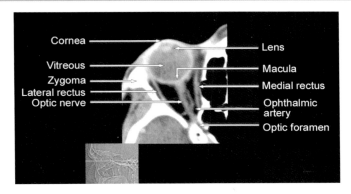

Figure 1.20: Axial CT section of right orbit

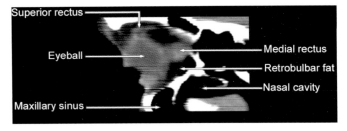

Figure 1.21: Sagittal CT recon of right orbit

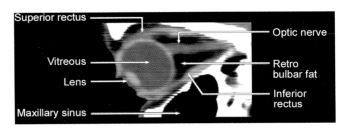

Figure 1.22: Sagittal CT recon of right orbit

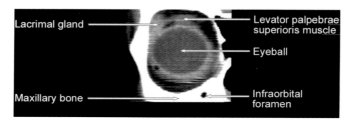

Lacrimal gland

Levator palpebrae superioris muscle

Eyeball

Maxillary bone

Infraorbital foramen

Figure 1.23: Coronal CT recon of right orbit

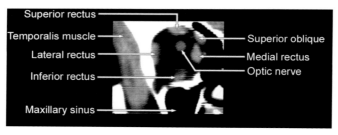

Superior rectus

Temporalis muscle

Lateral rectus

Inferior rectus

Maxillary sinus

Superior oblique

Medial rectus

Optic nerve

Figure 1.24: Coronal CT recon of right orbit

2 Temporal Bone

It has following portions:
1. Squamous
2. Mastoid
3. Petrous
4. Tympanic
5. Styloid

Ear is divided into external ear, middle ear and inner ear.

External ear has a bony and a cartilaginous external auditory canal and extends medially upto tympanic membrane.

Middle ear extends from tympanic membrane to the wall of bony labyrinth. It is divided into epitympanum, mesotympanum and hypotympanum by an upper line passing through inferior tip of scutum and a lower line drawn parallel to inferior aspect of bony external auditory canal. The auditory ossicles are: malleus, incus and stapes.

Inner ear includes the two and half turns of cochlea, vestibule, semicircular canals, cochlear aqueduct and vestibular aqueducts.

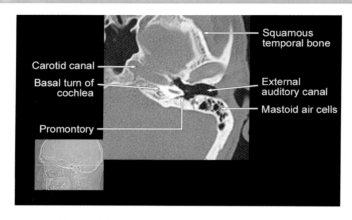

Figure 2.1: Axial CT section of left temporal bone

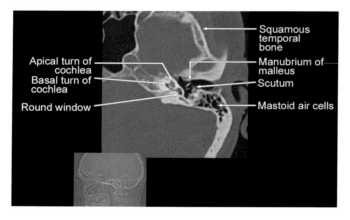

Figure 2.2: Axial CT section of left temporal bone

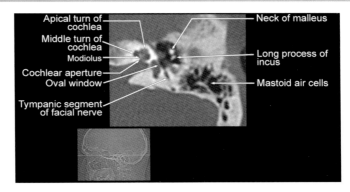

Figure 2.3: Axial CT section of left temporal bone

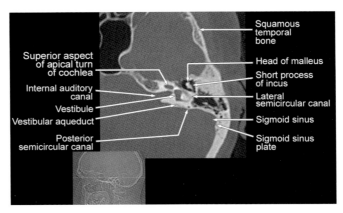

Figure 2.4: Axial CT section of left temporal bone

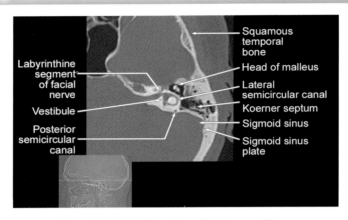

Figure 2.5: Axial CT section of left temporal bone

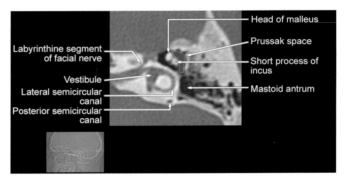

Figure 2.6: Axial CT section of left temporal bone magnified view

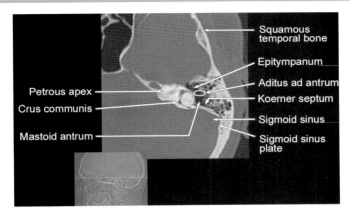

Figure 2.7: Axial CT section of left temporal bone

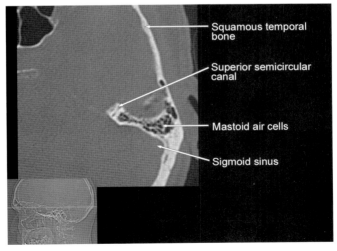

Figure 2.8: Axial CT section of left temporal bone

3 Paranasal Sinuses

Paranasal sinuses include maxillary sinuses, frontal sinus, anterior and posterior ethmoid sinuses and sphenoid sinus. They are lined with mucous membrane and communicate with nasal cavity.

Ostiomeatal unit is the common drainage for frontal, maxillary and anterior and middle ethmoid air cells into the nose. It produces two litres of mucus per day which travels towards nasopharynx at the rate of 1 cm/minute.

Certain variants of ethmoidal air cells are:

Onadi cells - pneumatized posterior most ethmoid air cells extending into sphenoid bone and optic canal.

Ethmoid bulla - air cell posterosuperior to infundibulum and lateral to lamina papyracea.

Haller cell is inferolateral to ethmoid bulla and protrudes into maxillary sinus.

Agger nasi is the anteriormost air cell in front of attachment of middle turbinate to cribriform plate.

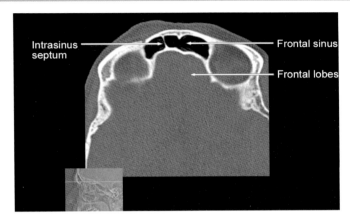

Figure 3.1: Axial CT section of PNS

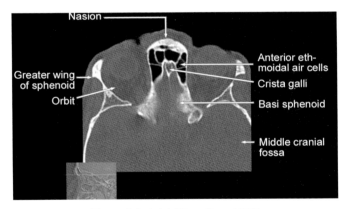

Figure 3.2: Axial CT section of PNS

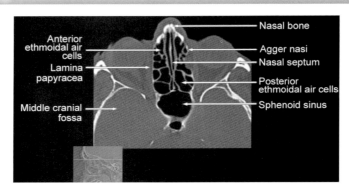

Figure 3.3: Axial CT section of PNS

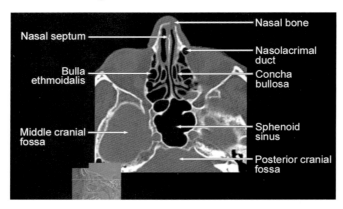

Figure 3.4: Axial CT section of PNS

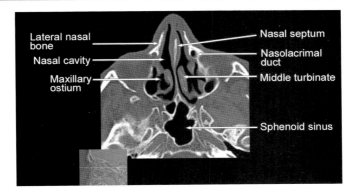

Figure 3.5: Axial CT section of PNS

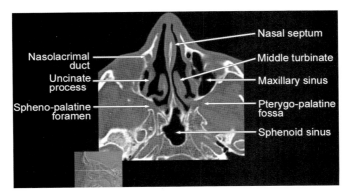

Figure 3.6: Axial CT section of PNS

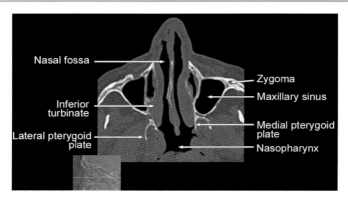

Figure 3.7: Axial CT section of PNS

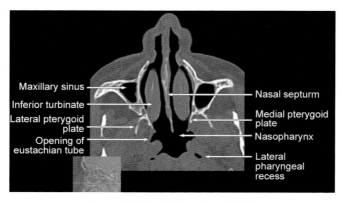

Figure 3.8: Axial CT section of PNS

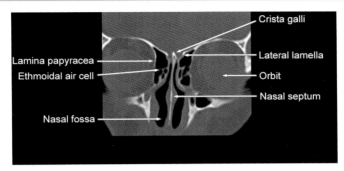

Figure 3.9: Coronal CT recon of PNS

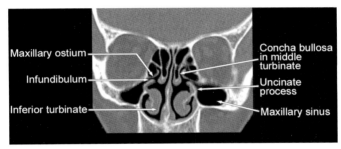

Figure 3.10: Coronal CT recon of PNS

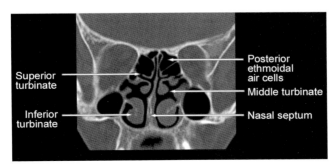

Figure 3.11: Coronal CT recon of PNS

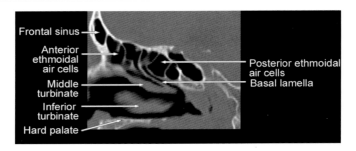

Figure 3.12: Sagittal CT recon of PNS

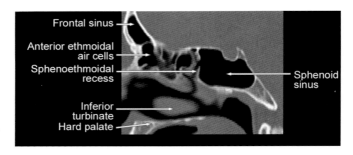

Figure 3.13: Sagittal CT recon of PNS

4 Face and Neck

Oral cavity includes lip, gingiva, buccal mucosa, hard palate, floor of mouth and anterior two thirds of tongue.

Oropharynx includes pharyngeal wall between nasopharynx and pharyngoepiglottic fold, soft palate, tonsillar region and tongue base.

Hypophayrnx is the aerodigestive tract between hyoid bone and inferior aspect of cricoid cartilage. It includes pyriform sinuses, pharyngoesophageal junction and posterior hypopharyngeal wall from valleculae to cricoarytenoid joints.

Larynx includes Supraglottic, Glottic and Subglottic compartments. Supraglottic compartment is from tongue base and valleculae to laryngeal ventricle. Glottis includes the true vocal cord along with anterior and posterior commissure. Subglottis extends from undersurface of true vocal cords to cricoid.

Deep Spaces of Suprahyoid Portion of Neck are:
1. Masticator space
2. Pharyngeal mucosal space
3. Parapharyngeal space
4. Retropharyngeal space
5. Prevertebral space
6. Carotid space
7. Parotid space
8. Submandibular space

Salivary Glands

There are three pairs of salivary glands: the parotids, the sub-mandibular and the sublingual glands.

Parotid gland is located in the parotid space at the angle of mandible. It has a superficial lobe (which forms the main bulk), deep lobe and an accessory lobe. It is drained by Stenson's duct that opens opposite the upper second molar tooth.

Thyroid gland appears slightly hyperdense on CT scan and has a value of 60-120 HU.

Parathyroid glands are four in number. Two superior para-thyroid and two inferior parathyroid glands. Rarely supernumerary parathyroid glands can be seen between 6-12 in number.

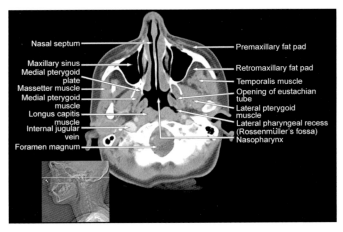

Figure 4.1: Axial CT section of neck

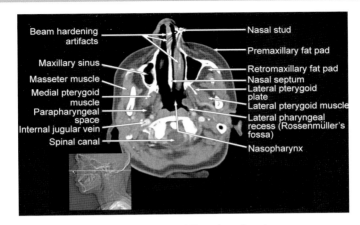

Figure 4.2: Axial CT section of neck

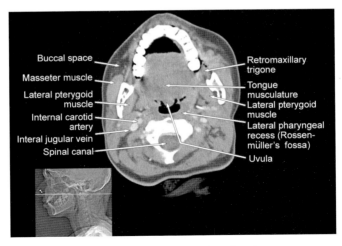

Figure 4.3: Axial CT section of neck

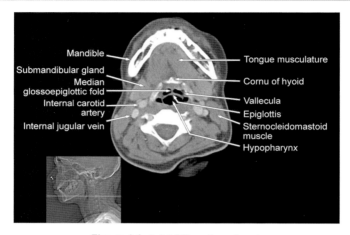

Figure 4.4: Axial CT section of neck

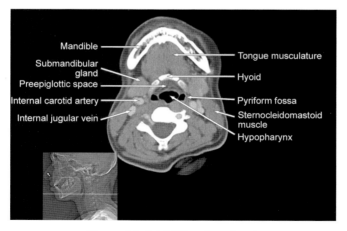

Figure 4.5: Axial CT section of neck

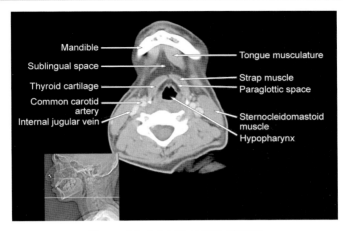

Figure 4.6: Axial CT section of neck

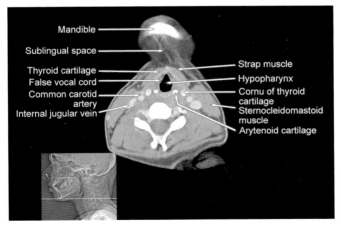

Figure 4.7: Axial CT section of neck

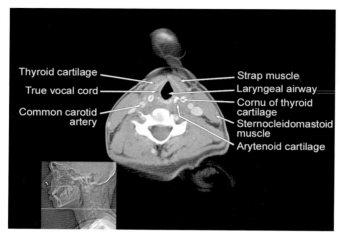

Figure 4.8: Axial CT section of neck

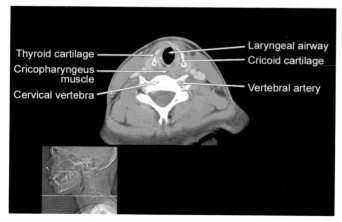

Figure 4.9: Axial CT section of neck

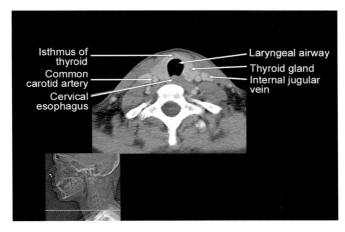

Figure 4.10: Axial CT section of neck

5 Vertebral Column

It is formed by 33 bones called vertebrae which are connected with each other by joints and have a cushion of intervertebral disc in between. A typical vertebra has a body, pedicle anteriorly, transverse process laterally, lamina posterolaterally and spinous process posteriorly. Vertebral column is made of cervical, thoracic, lumbar, sacral and coccygeal vertebrae.

1. Anterior column is formed by anterior longitudinal ligament, anterior annulus fibrosus and anterior part of vertebral body.
2. Middle column is formed by posterior longitudinal ligament, posterior annulus fibrosus and posterior part of vertebral body.
3. Posterior column includes posterior elements and ligaments.

Craniovertebral Junction

Chamberlain line is the line between posterior part of hard palate and posterior margin of foramen magnum. Normally the tip of Odontoid process lies at or below this line.

Basilar line is the line along the clivus and it usually falls tangent to posterior aspect of tip of Odontoid.

Craniovertebral angle (Clivus-Canal angle) is angle between basilar line and a line along posterior aspect of odontoid process. If this angle is $< 150°$, cord compression can occur on the ventral aspect.

Coverings of Spinal Cord

1. Periosteum is formed by continuation of outer layer of cerebral dura mater.

2. Epidural space is between dura mater and bone and contains epidural veins, lymphatic, fat and connective tissues.
3. Dura mater is the continuation of inner layer of cerebral dura mater and ends at second lumbar vertebral level. It sends extensions around spinal nerves and continues with epineurium of peripheral nerves.
4. Subarachnoid space extends between arachnoid and pia mater. It contains CSF.
5. Pia mater is firmly adherent to spinal cord.

Vertebral Canal

If the conus medullaris is at or below L3 vertebral level rule out tethering of cord, bony spur or thick filum.

1. Axial CT images of occipital condyles/base of skull (Fig. 5.1), C1 vertebra/Atlas (Figs 5.2 and 5.3) C2 vertebra/Axis (Figs 5.4 and 5.5).
2. Coronal CT images of Atlanto-occipital and Atlanto-axial junction (Fig. 5.6).
3. Axial CT image of typical cervical vertebra (Fig. 5.7)
4. Volume rendered CT images C1-C2 level; axial view (Fig. 5.8), Coronal view (Fig. 5.9) and Sagittal view (Fig. 5.10).
5. Volume rendered CT images of other cervical vertebrae; axial view (Fig. 5.11), coronal view (Fig. 5.12) and sagittal view (Fig. 5.13).
6. Axial CT image of typical thoracic vertebra (Fig. 5.14).
7. Coronal CT image of thoraco-lumbar junction (Fig. 5.15).
8. Volume rendered CT images of thoracic spine; coronal view (Fig. 5.16) and sagittal view (Fig. 5.17).
9. Axial CT images of typical lumbar vertebra (Fig. 5.18) and Sacroiliac region (Fig. 5.19).
10. Coronal CT image of lumbo-sacral region (Fig. 5.20).

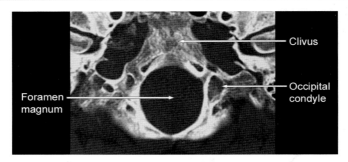

Figure 5.1: Occipital condyle

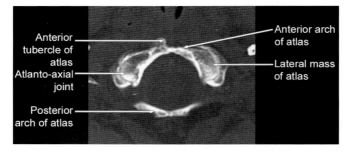

Figure 5.2: C1 vertebra (atlas)

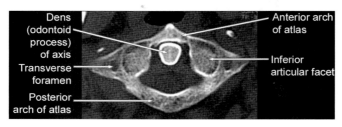

Figure 5.3: C1 vertebra

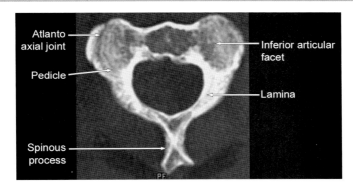

Figure 5.4: C2 vertebra

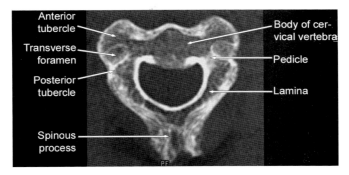

Figure 5.5: C2 vertebra

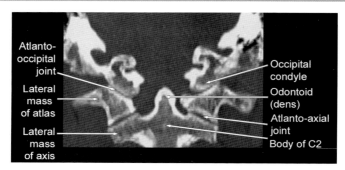

Figure 5.6: C1-C2 coronal recon

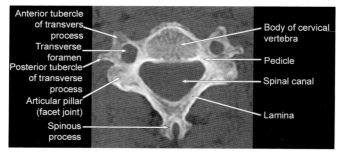

Figure 5.7: Typical cervical vertebra (C3-C7)

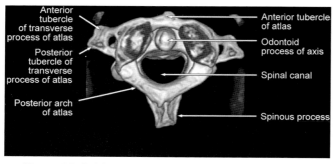

Figure 5.8: Axial view (C1-C2 level) volume rendered image

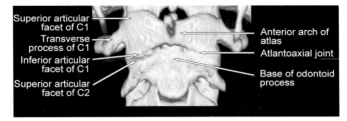

Figure 5.9: Coronal view (C1-C2 level) volume rendered image

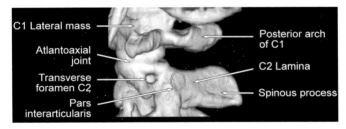

Figure 5.10: Sagittal view (C1-C2 level) volume rendered image

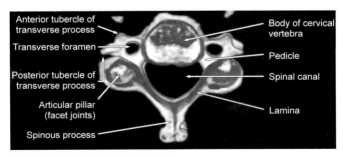

Figure 5.11: Axial typical vertebra (C3-C7) volume rendered image

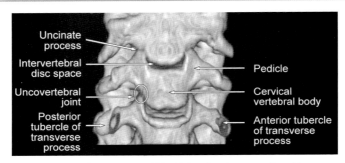

Figure 5.12: Coronal view (C2-C4 level) volume rendered image

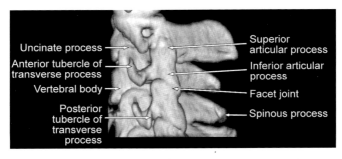

Figure 5.13: Sagittal view (C2-C4 level) volume rendered image

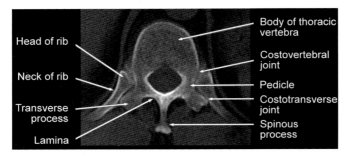

Figure 5.14: Typical thoracic vertebra

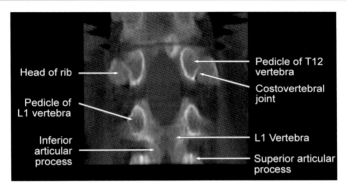

Figure 5.15: T12-L1 coronal

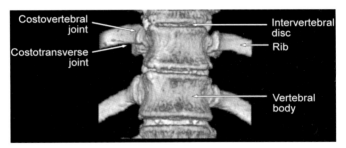

Figure 5.16: Coronal view (Typical thoracic vertebrae)

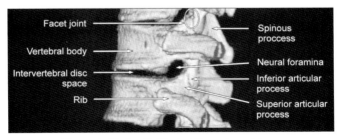

Figure 5.17: Sagittal typical thoracic vertebrae

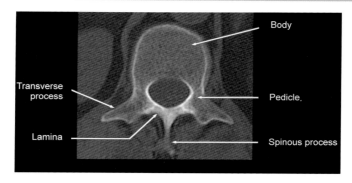

Figure 5.18: Typical lumbar vertebra

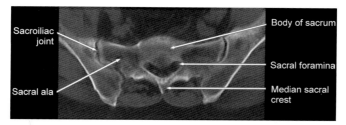

Figure 5.19: S1 vertebra and sacroiliac joints

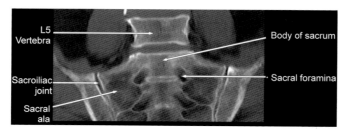

Figure 5.20: L5-S1 coronal recon

6 Chest and Mediastinum

Embryologically airway starts developing by fifth week of gestational age in the form of lung buds which grow from ventral aspect of primitive foregut. Trachea and esophagus are also separated by fifth week. Hereafter tracheobronchial tree is formed from fifth to fifteenth week. There are 23-25 airway generations from trachea to bronchiole. Bronchus has cartilage in the wall, whereas bronchiole is devoid of cartilage.

Interstitium of lung is divided into axial interstitium, parenchymal interstitial interstitium and peripheral interstitium. Axial interstitium is made of bronchovascular sheaths and lymphatics. Parenchymal interstitium includes interalveolar septum along alveolar walls. Peripheral interstitium includes sub-pleural connective tissue and interlobular septa which encloses the pulmonary veins and lymphatics.

Pulmonary circulation includes primary pulmonary circulation, bronchial circulation and the anastomoses between the two. Primary pulmonary circulation consists of pulmonary arteries and veins that travel down to sub-segmental bronchial level and has a diameter same as that of the accompanying airway. Main pulmonary artery arises from the right ventricle.

Bronchial circulation originates from thoracic aorta and supplies through the intercostal arteries which are two in number for each lung.

Segmental division of lungs:

Right lung has three lobes:

1. Upper lobe which has an apical, anterior and a posterior segment.
2. Middle lobe has a lateral and a medial segment.
3. Lower lobe has superior segment, medial basal segment, anterior basal segment, lateral basal segment and a posterior basal segment.

Left lung has two lobes:

1. Upper lobe which has an apico-posterior, anterior, superior lingular and an inferior lingular segment.
2. Lower lobe has superior segment, anterior basal segment, lateral basal segment and a posterior basal segment.

Left lung has no middle lobe.

Mediastinum is the space between the lungs. It is divided into a superior and an inferior compartment. Superior compartment consists of the thoracic inlet. Inferior compartment has anterior, middle and posterior subcompartments. Retrosternal region is included in the anterior compartment, heart lies in the middle compartment and descending aorta with esophagus and paraspinal region is located in the posterior mediastinal compartment. Thymus is located in the anterior part of superior as well as inferior compartment of mediastinum.

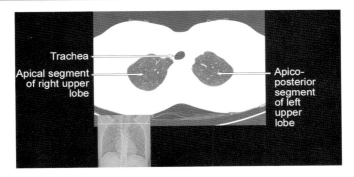

Figure 6.1

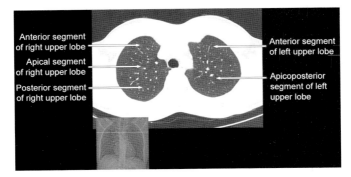

Figure 6.2

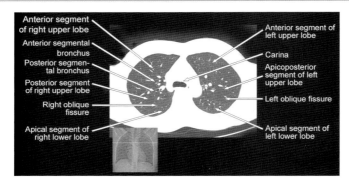

Figure 6.3

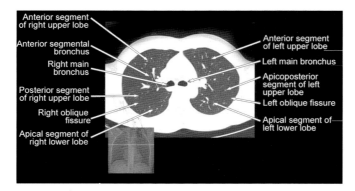

Figure 6.4

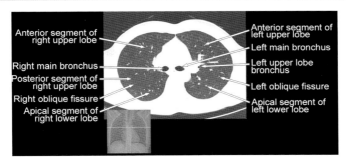

Figure 6.5

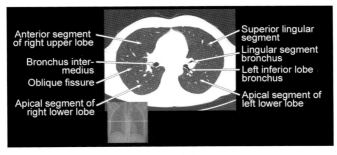

Figure 6.6

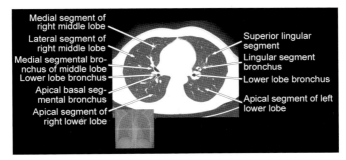

Figure 6.7

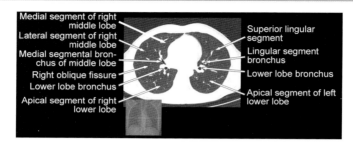

Figure 6.8

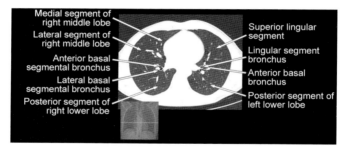

Figure 6.9

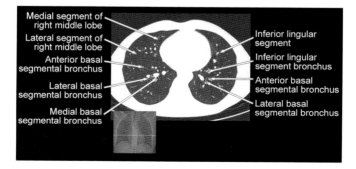

Figure 6.10

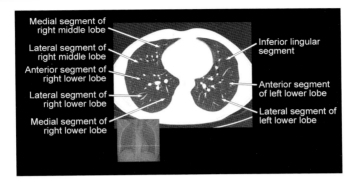

Figure 6.11

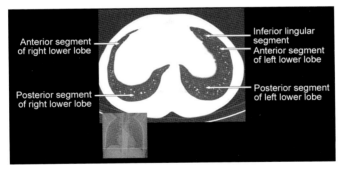

Figure 6.12

Figures 6.1 to 6.12: Axial CT section of lungs

CT MEDIASTINUM

NORMAL ANATOMY

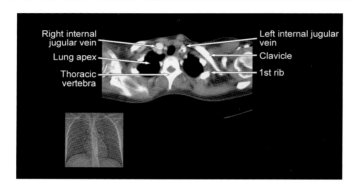

Figure 6.13

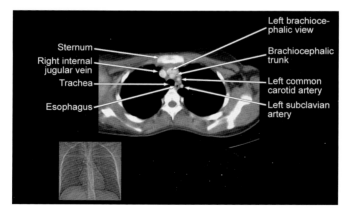

Figure 6.14

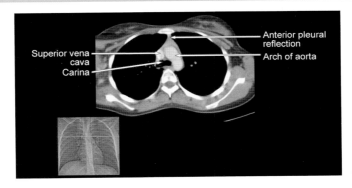

Figure 6.15

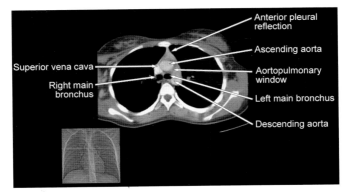

Figure 6.16

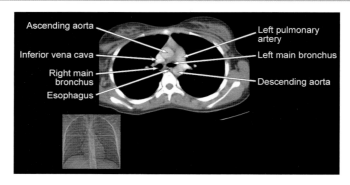

Figure 6.17

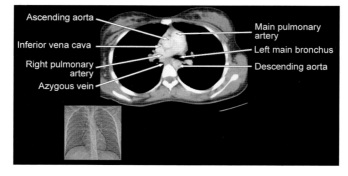

Figure 6.18

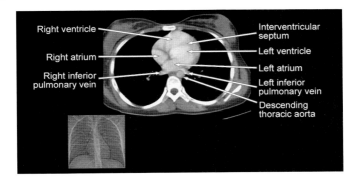

Figure 6.19

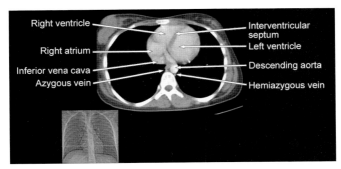

Figure 6.20

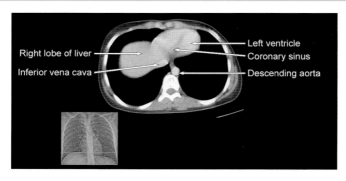

Figure 6.21

7 Heart

CT CORONARY ANGIOGRAPHY
NORMAL ANATOMY

Heart imaging methods such as cardiac CT are allowing physicians to take a closer look at the heart and great vessels at little risk to the patient.

A traditional CT scan is an X-ray procedure which combines many X-ray images with the aid of a computer to generate cross-sectional views of the body. Cardiac CT uses advanced CT technology with or without intravenous iodine-based contrast to visualize cardiac anatomy, including the coronary arteries and great arteries and veins. With multi-detector scanning, it is possible to acquire high-resolution three-dimensional images of the heart and great vessels.

Cardiac CT is especially useful in evaluating the myocardium, coronary arteries, pulmonary veins, thoracic aorta, pericardium, and cardiac masses, such as thrombus of the left atrial appendage.

Coronary Arteries

The four main coronary arteries evaluated by CT are the right coronary artery (RCA), the left main coronary artery (LCA), the left anterior descending (LAD) artery, and the left circumflex (LCx) artery.

Dominant Coronary Artery

Whichever artery crosses the crux of the heart and gives off the posterior descending branches is considered to be the dominant coronary artery.

In approximately 85% of individuals, the RCA crosses the posterior interventricular groove and gives rise to the posterior descending branches (right dominance); in 7-8%, the LCx artery crosses the interventricular groove and gives rise to branches to the posterior right ventricular surface (left dominance); and in the remaining 7-8%, the inferior interventricular septum is perfused by branches from both the distal RCA and the distal LCx artery (co-dominance).

Right Coronary Artery: The RCA arises from the anterior right coronary sinus somewhat inferior to the origin of the LCA. The RCA passes to the right of and posterior to the pulmonary artery and then downward in the right atrioventricular groove toward the posterior interventricular septum.

In more than 50% of individuals, the first branch of the RCA is the conus artery, unless it (the RCA) has a separate origin directly from the right coronary sinus.

The second branches usually consist of the sinoatrial node/ nodal artery and several anterior branches that supply the free wall of the right ventricle.

The branch to the right ventricle at the junction of the middle and distal RCA is called the acute marginal branch.

The distal RCA divides into posterior descending artery (PDA) and posterior left ventricular branches (PLV) in a right dominant anatomy.

Left Coronary Artery: The LCA arises from the left posterior coronary sinus and is 5-10 mm long. The LCA passes to the left of and posterior to the pulmonary trunk and bifurcates into the LAD and LCx arteries. Occasionally, the LCA trifurcates into the LAD and LCx arteries and the ramus intermedius. The ramus intermedius has a course similar to that of the first diagonal branch of the LAD artery to the anterior left ventricle.

The LAD artery passes to the left of the pulmonary trunk and turns anteriorly to course in the anterior interventricular groove toward the apex. It provides the diagonal branches (D) to the anterior free wall of the left ventricle and the septal branches to the anterior interventricular septum.

The Left Circumflex Artery (LCx) courses in the left atrioventricular groove and gives off Obtuse Marginal branches (OM) to the lateral left ventricle.

In a left dominant or codominant anatomy, the LCx artery gives rise to the PDA or posterior left ventricular branches.

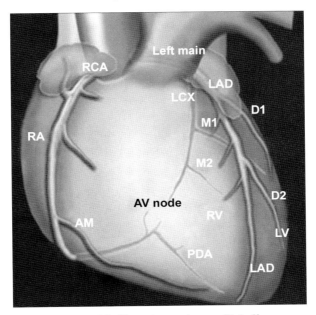

Figure 7.1: *(For color version see Plate 2)*

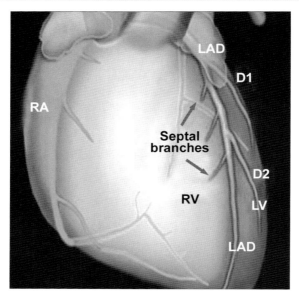

Figure 7.2: *(For color version see Plate 3)*

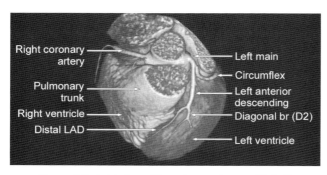

Figure 7.3: Axial plane *(For color version see Plate 3)*

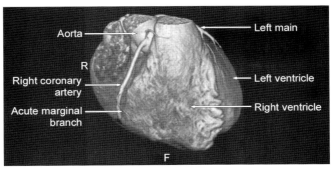

Figure 7.4: Coronal plane *(For color version see Plate 4)*

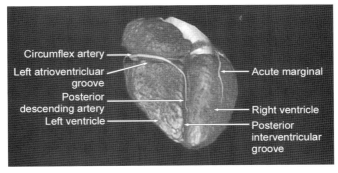

Figure 7.5: Posterior coronal plane *(For color version see Plate 4)*

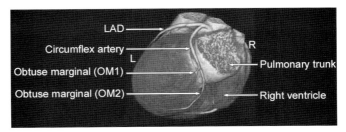

Figure 7.6: Posterior oblique coronal plane *(For color version see Plate 4)*

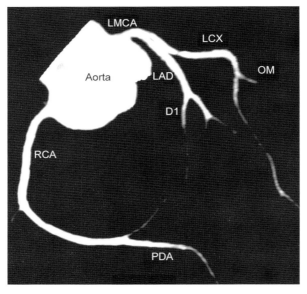

Figure 7.7: Coronal plane (MIP image)

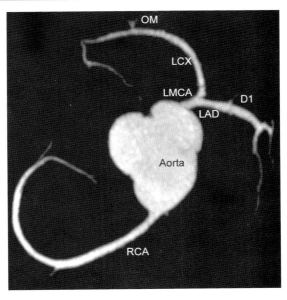

Figure 7.8: Axial plane (MIP image)

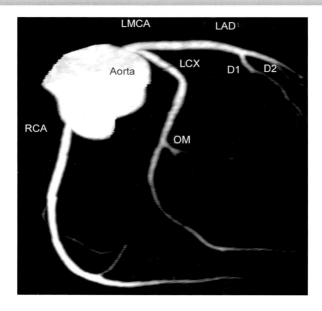

Figure 7.9: Oblique coronal plane

8 Abdomen and Pelvis

LIVER

Functional segmental anatomy of liver is based on distribution of three hepatic veins. Middle hepatic vein divides the liver into right and left lobes. Left hepatic vein divides the left lobe into medial and lateral parts. Right hepatic vein divides the right lobe into the anterior and posterior parts. An imaginary transverse line through the right and left portal vein divides these parts into anterior and posterior segments which are numbered counterclockwise from the Inferior Vena Cava.

The Couinaud classification of liver anatomy divides the liver into eight functionally indepedent segments. Each segment has its own vascular inflow, outflow and biliary drainage. In the centre of each segment there is a branch of the portal vein, hepatic artery and bile duct. The numbering of the segments is in a clockwise manner.

Segment 1 (caudate lobe) is located posteriorly and extends between fissure of the ligamentum venosum anteriorly and the inferior venacava posteriorly.

The longitudinal plane of the right hepatic vein divides segment 8 from segment 7 in the superior portion of the liver and in the inferior portion of the liver segment 5 from segment 6.

The longitudinal plane of the middle hepatic vein through the gallbladder fossa separates segment 4a from segment 8 in the superior liver and segment 4b from segment 5 in the inferior liver.

The longitudinal plane of the left hepatic vein and fissure of the ligamentum teres separates segment 4a from segment 2 in the superior liver and segment 4b from segment 3 in the inferior liver.

The axial plane of the left portal vein separates segment 4a superiorly from segment 4b inferiorly and segment 2 superiorly from segment 3 inferiorly in the left lobe.

The axial plane of the right portal vein separates segment 8 and segment 7 superiorly from segment 5 and segment 6 inferiorly in the right lobe.

Normal liver has a precontrast attenuation value of 45-65 H.U. and maximum enhancement occurs at 50-60 seconds after administration of contrast. Normal liver has a size upto 13 centimeters. Normal portal vein is 10-13 mm in diameter.

GALLBLADDER

Normal gallbladder is upto 10 cm long and 4 cm wide. It has a normal wall thickness upto 3 mm. Gallbladder may have septae. Bifid appearance is due to longitudinal septum. Phrygian cap gall bladder is due to kink or septum at the neck. Ectopic gallbladder can be seen beneath the left lobe of liver or even in retro hepatic location. Floating gallbladder can result from loose peritoneal attachments.

Normal cystic duct is 2 cm long and 2 mm wide. Maximum diameter of normal common bile duct in an adult is 2-5 mm. Post cholecystectomy it can be upto 7 mm. Normal width increases by 1mm per decade in elderly over 60 years of age.

PANCREAS

It develops during the fourth week of gestation as the second endodermal diverticulum from foregut. The dorsal diverticulum forms the dorsal pancreas. Ventral diverticulum forms the ventral pancreas as well as the liver, gallbladder and bile ducts.

The main pancreatic duct is known as the duct of Wirsung. The angle between the pancreatic duct and common bile duct at their joining point is between 5 to 30°. These ducts open into second part of duodenum through the ampulla of Vater which has a sphincter called the sphincter of Oddi.

The entire length of pancreas is 10-15 cm. Pancreatic tail is upto 1.6 cm thick; body is upto 1.1 cm thick and the head ranges from 1-2 cm in thickness.

Annular pancreas is a congenital anomaly in which the duodenum is enclosed on all sides by pancreas as a result of abnormal migration of ventral pancreas.

SPLEEN

Spleen is formed during fifth week of gestational age from mesenchymal cells between layers of dorsal mesogastrium. Accessory spleen can be seen in 10-30 % of patients. Spleen can even be attached to left testis or ovary as there is a close relationship between the left gonadal anlage and the splenic precursor mesenchymal cells (Spleno-gonadal fusion). It has a weight upto 200 gm and a length of 11 cm. The CT value of spleen is 5 HU less than the liver.

THE GASTROINTESTINAL SYSTEM

The gastrointestinal system originates from a pouch like extension of yolk sac starting from 6 weeks of gestational age. The foregut is supplied by celiac artery, midgut by superior mesenteric artery and the hindgut by inferior mesenteric artery.

Upper gastrointestinal system starts from mouth and continues into oropharynx which continues into esophagus. Esophagus is a 25 cm long tubular structure which opens into the stomach via gastro esophageal junction. Parts of stomach are the fundus, body, greater and lesser curvatures, antrum and pylorus. Walls are 3-5 mm thick except in pylorus where it can be upto 7 mm thick.

Small intestine can be upto 6 m long and extends from pyloric orifice of stomach upto ileocaecal valve. Duodenum is 1 feet long, jejunum is around 10 feet and ileum is upto 8 feet. Fifteen centimeters long mesentery is located between ileocaecal junction and ligament of Treitz. Circular folds of small bowel are called as valvulae conniventes.

Rule of three for normal small bowel states that its walls are 3 mm thick, valvulae conniventes are 3 mm thick, there are less than 3 air fluid levels and the diameter is upto 3 cm.

Large intestine is 1.5 m long and extends from ileum to anus. Its parts are caecum, ascending colon, hepatic flexure of colon, transverse colon, splenic flexure, descending colon, sigmoid colon, rectum and anal canal.

Peritoneal spaces above transverse colon are

I. Spaces on the right
    1. Right subphrenic space
    2. Anterior and posterior right sub hepatic space
    3. Bare area of liver
    4. Lesser sac
II. Spaces on the left
    1. Left subphrenic space
    2. Left sub hepatic space
    3. Perisplenic space

Peritoneal Spaces below transverse colon are

1. Superior and Inferior Ileocecal recesses
2. Retrocecal space
3. Right and left paracolic gutters
4. Intersigmoid recess

Two folds of peritoneum supporting a structure within the peritoneal cavity together form a structure known as ligament.

When two folds of peritoneum connect a portion of bowel to the retroperitoneum it is known as mesentery. Ventral mesentery gives rise to falciform ligament, gastrohepatic ligament and hepatoduodenal ligament. Dorsal mesentery gives rise to gastro-phrenic ligament, gastropancreatic ligament, phrenicocolic ligament, gastrosplenic ligament, splenorenal ligament and gastrocolic ligament. Dorsal mesentery also forms the small bowel mesentery and transverse as well as sigmoid mesocolons.

Omentum is a structure connecting stomach to an additional structure. Lesser omentum is formed by combination of hepatoduodenal and gastro hepatic ligament. Greater omentum is an inferior continuation of gastro colic ligament and is composed of four layers of peritoneum resulting from double reflection of dorsal mesogastrium.

Anterior right subhepatic space located posterior to porta hepatis communicates with lesser sac through epiploic foramen also known as foramen of Winslow.

UROGENITAL SYSTEM

- Kidneys arise from metanephros (of mesodermal origin) at fourth week of intrauterine life. Bladder, Urethra and prostate are formed from urogenital sinus.
- Adult kidneys have a span of 7-12 cm. Renal arteries arise from abdominal aorta at the level of L1-L2 vertebrae and then divide into following five segmental branches: apical, anterior superior, anterior inferior, posterior and basilar.
- Renal arteries can be multiple, aberrant, accessory and even supplementary. Single or multiple renal veins can exist.
- Retroperitoneum is the space between parietal peritoneum extending from diaphragm to pelvic brim and fascia transversalis.
- Adrenal glands (suprarenal glands) are situated on the top of kidneys and are 3cm long and 1 cm thick.
- Average size of testis is $2.5 \times 3.0 \times 3.5$ cm. Epididymis has a head, body and a tail.
- Spermatic cord consists of testicular artery, cremasteric artery, pampaniform plexus of veins, vas deferens, nerves and lymphatics.
- Gonadal artery arises from ventral surface of aorta slightly below the origin of renal arteries. Occasionally it can arise from renal artery.

- Gonadal veins drain in the IVC or renal vein on right and in the renal vein on left.
- Prostate has a normal size of $2.5 \times 2.8 \times 3.0$ cm. It is composed of an outer part having a central and peripheral zone and an inner part made of periurethral and transitional zone.
- Male urethra is 15-20 cm long and has a posterior part composed of prostatic urethra and membranous urethra. The anterior part of urethra is composed of bulbar and penile urethra.

Female urethra is 2.5-5 cm long.

Adult Uterus is 6-9cm long, 2.5-4 cm anteroposterior and 3-4.5 cm transverse in dimension. Endometrium is the innermost zone of uterus. Serosa is the outermost zone. Myometrium is the middle layer. CT scan usually does not show them separately.

Fallopian tubes arise from upper and the outer aspect of uterus, and extend between the folds of broad ligament towards the pelvic side walls to open just above and anterior to ovaries located in ovarian fossa on each side.

Pelvic spaces formed due to relationship between urinary bladder, uterus and rectum are:
1. Recto uterine pouch of Douglas
2. Uterovesicle pouch
3. Recto vesicle recess
   Important Pelvic ligaments in relation to uterus are:
1. Broad ligament - between uterus and pelvic sidewalls
2. Round ligament – between uterus and labia majora
3. Cardinal ligament/Mackenrodt ligament - between cervix and fascia of obturator internus
4. Uterosacral ligament – between uterus and sacrum
   Adult ovaries measure 0.5-1.5 cm $\times$ 1.5-3.0 cm $\times$ 2-3 cm.

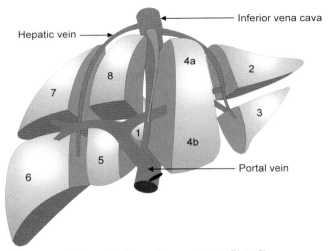

Figure 8.1 (For color version see Plate 5)

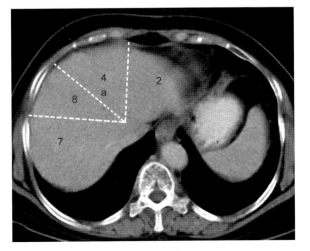

Figure 8.2

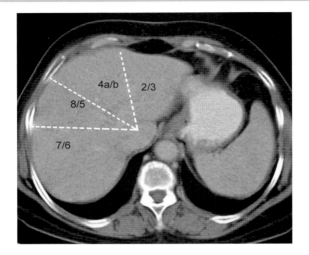

Figure 8.3

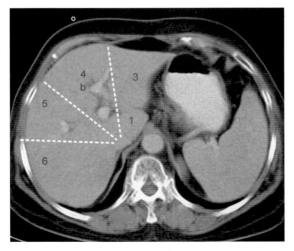

Figure 8.4

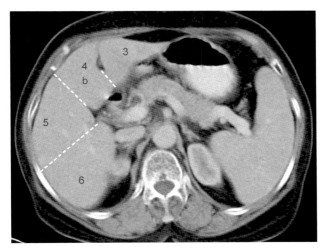

Figure 8.5

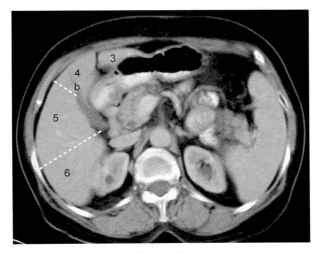

Figure 8.6

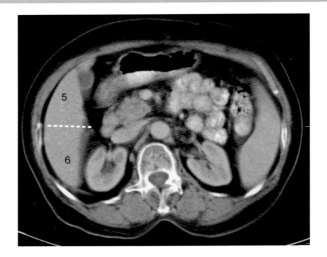

Figure 8.7

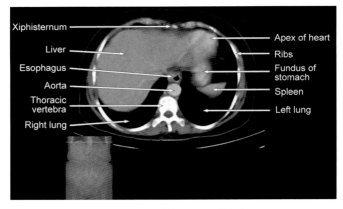

Figure 8.8: Axial CT section of abdomen

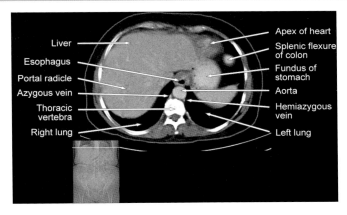

Figure 8.9: Axial CT section of abdomen

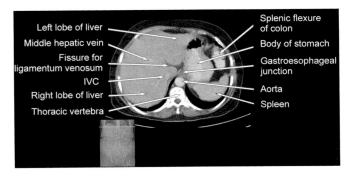

Figure 8.10: Axial CT section of abdomen

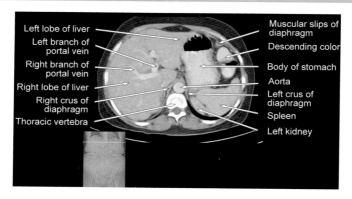

Figure 8.11: Axial CT section of abdomen

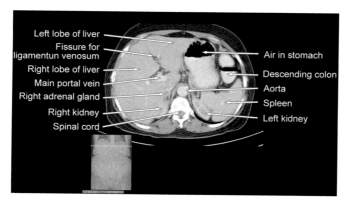

Figure 8.12: Axial CT section of abdomen

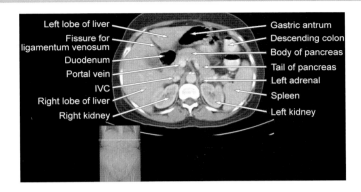

Figure 8.13: Axial CT section of abdomen

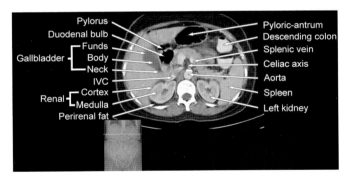

Figure 8.14: Axial CT section of abdomen

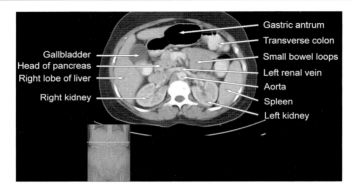

Figure 8.15: Axial CT section of abdomen

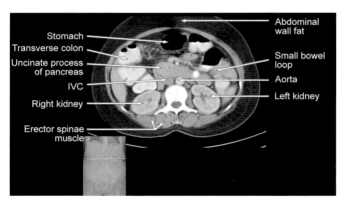

Figure 8.16: Axial CT section of abdomen

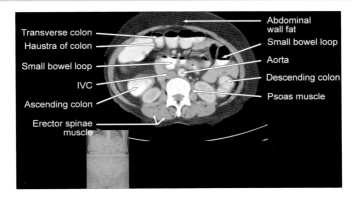

Figure 8.17: Axial CT section of abdomen

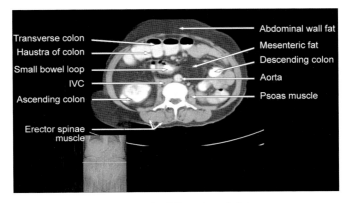

Figure 8.18: Axial CT section of abdomen

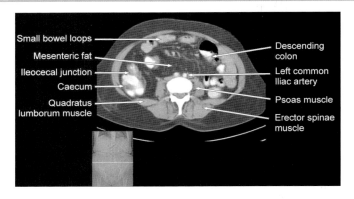

Figure 8.19: Axial CT section of abdomen

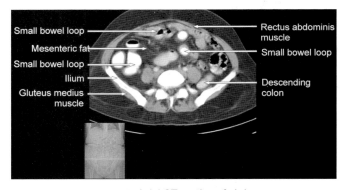

Figure 8.20: Axial CT section of abdomen

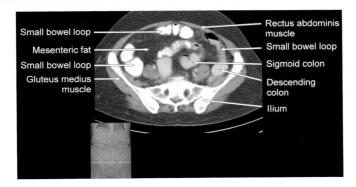

Figure 8.21: Axial CT section of abdomen

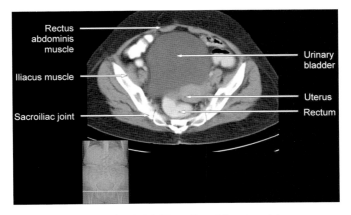

Figure 8.22: Axial CT section of female pelvis

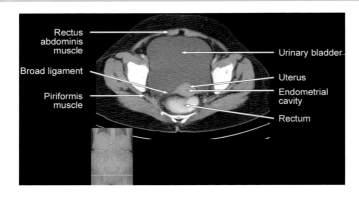

Figure 8.23: Axial CT section of female pelvis

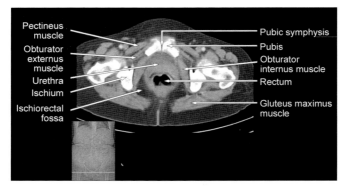

Figure 8.24: Axial CT section of female pelvis

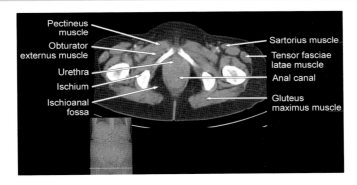

Figure 8.25: Axial CT section of female pelvis

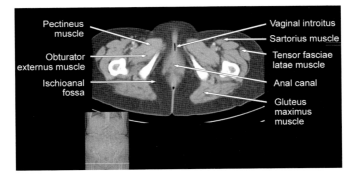

Figure 8.26: Axial CT section of female pelvis

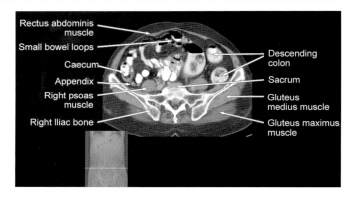

Figure 8.27: Axial CT section showing appendix

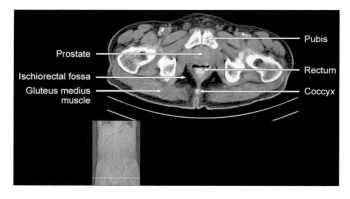

Figure 8.28: Axial CT section of male pelvis

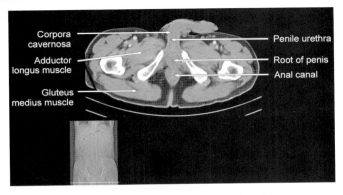

Figure 8.29: Axial CT section of male pelvis

Joints of Upper Extremity

It has three parts:

a. Upper arm which has a bone: humerus.
b. Forearm which has two bones: radius and ulna
c. Wrist and Hand: Wrist has 8 carpals and hand has 5 metacarpals and 14 phalanges.

The upper limb is attached to the trunk by shoulder girdle which is made of scapula posteriorly and clavicle anteriorly.

SHOULDER JOINT

It is a ball and socket type synovial joint formed by glenoid of scapula and head of humerus. Humeral head is large and broad than glenoid cavity due to which this joint is intrinsically weak. Hence to provide stability to this joint, it is surrounded by rotator cuff made of muscles and tendons and coracoacromial arch made of coracoid process, acromian, coracoacromial ligament and acromioclavicular joint. Strong superior, middle and inferior gleno-humeral capsular ligaments also impart glenohumeral stabity.

Rotator cuff is formed by subscapularis, supraspinatus, infraspinatus and teres minor arranged antero-posteriorly.

Complex intra-articular fractures and fractures of scapula can particularly be seen in great details by CT scan.

ELBOW JOINT

Distal articulating surface of humerus and proximal articulating surfaces of radius and ulna participate in forming this synovial joint. Radial head is aligned in place against radial notch of ulna by annular ligament. Radial collateral ligament and ulnar collateral ligament also help keeping elbow in reduction. Triceps is the main extensor and biceps is the main supinator of elbow.

CT is particularly useful in detecting subtle fractures, loose bodies and the extent of heterotopic bone formation in and around elbow joint.

WRIST JOINT

Radio-carpal and distal radio-ulnar joints together form the wrist joint. Subtle fractures and dislocations of carpals like scaphoid and lunate and distal radio-ulnar dislocations are best seen on CT scan even though plain radiographs may appear normal. Persistent pain on radial aspect of palm particularly in golfers is usually due to fracture of hook of hamate and is best shown by CT scan.

CT SHOULDER

NORMAL ANATOMY

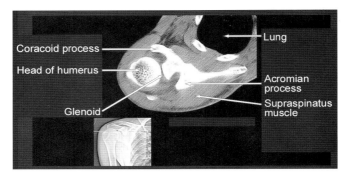

Figure 9.1: Axial CT section of shoulder

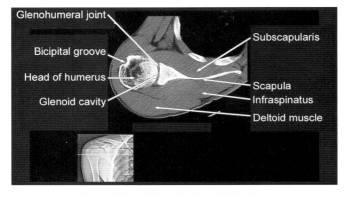

Figure 9.2: Axial CT section of shoulder

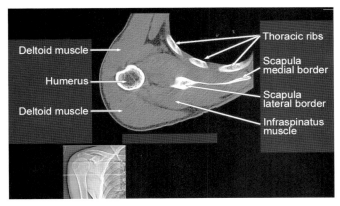

Figure 9.3: Axial CT section of shoulder

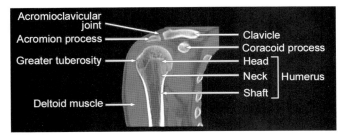

Figure 9.4: Coronal recon of shoulder

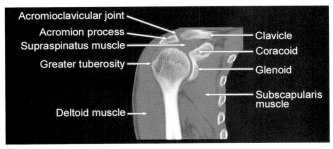

Figure 9.5: Coronal recon of shoulder

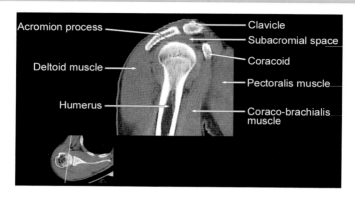

Figure 9.6: Sagittal recon of shoulder

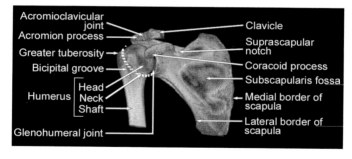

Figure 9.7: Volume rendered recon of shoulder
(Anteroposterior projection)

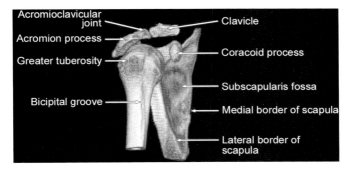

Figure 9.8: Volume rendered recon of shoulder
(Lateral oblique projection)

CT ELBOW JOINT

NORMAL ANATOMY

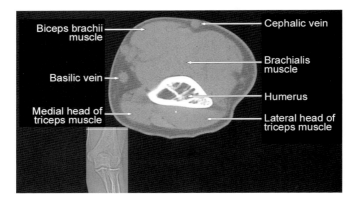

Figure 9.9: Axial CT section of elbow

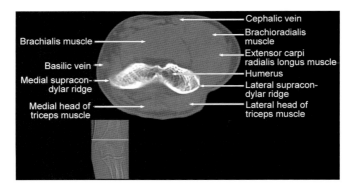

Figure 9.10: Axial CT section of elbow

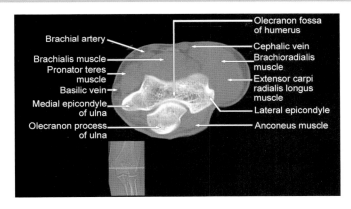

Figure 9.11: Axial CT section of elbow

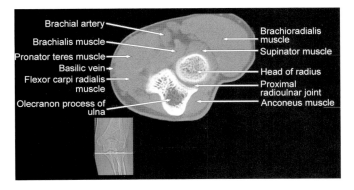

Figure 9.12: Axial CT section of elbow

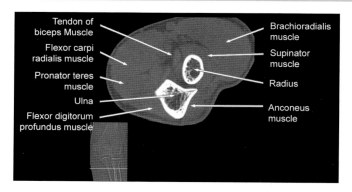

Figure 9.13: Axial CT section of elbow

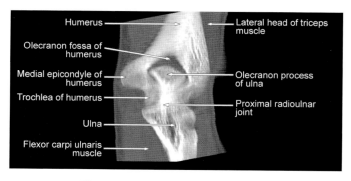

Figure 9.14: Coronal CT recon of elbow

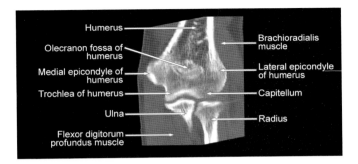

Figure 9.15: Coronal CT recon of elbow

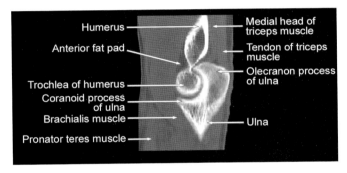

Figure 9.16: Sagittal CT recon of elbow

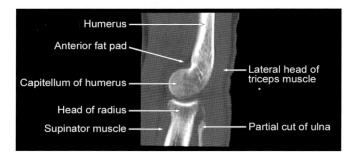

Figure 9.17: Sagittal CT recon of elbow

CT WRIST

NORMAL ANATOMY

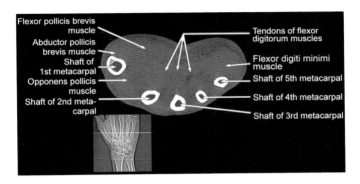

Figure 9.18: Axial CT section of wrist

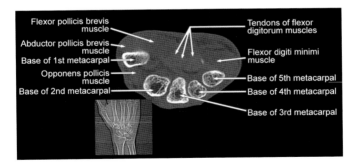

Figure 9.19: Axial CT section of wrist

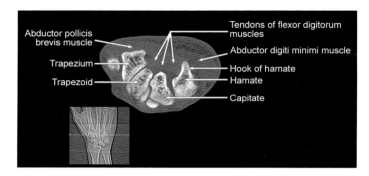

Figure 9.20: Axial CT section of wrist

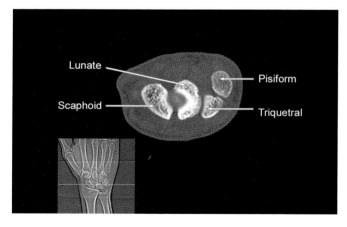

Figure 9.21: Axial CT section of wrist

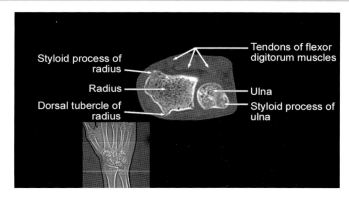

Figure 9.22: Axial CT section of wrist

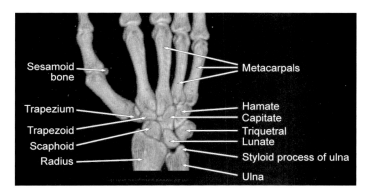

Figure 9.23: Volume rendered recon of wrist

10 Joints of Lower Extremity

It has three parts:

a. Thigh which has a bone called femur which is the longest and strongest bone in the body.

b. Leg has two bones known as tibia and fibula.

c. Ankle and Feet. Ankle has 7 tarsals. Feet have 5 metatarsals and 14 phalanges.

The pelvis is a ring of bones situated between lower part of vertebral column and the lower limb. Posteriorly it is formed by sacrum and anterolaterally by two hip bones. Each hip bone has three portions called as ilium, ischium and pubis.

HIP JOINT

It is a complex ball and socket type synovial joint formed by femoral head, acetabulum, soft tissues, muscles and cartilages. CT scan of hip joint followed by reformations in various planes provides exquisite details in multiple planes for an ideal three dimensional perspective. Complex acetabular fractures and loose bodies or bone fragments are best seen on CT scan.

KNEE JOINT

Distal articulating surface of femur and proximal articulating surfaces of tibia and fibula participate in forming this synovial joint. The tibio-femoral articulation is the main component of knee joint and is made stable by anterior and posterior cruciate ligaments and medial and lateral collateral ligaments. Joint surfaces are separated by medial and lateral menisci for shock absorption. Patello-femoral articulation imparts better leverage to quadriceps movement thereby further strengthening it.

Complex multiplanar fractures and loose bodies are best seen by CT scan.

THE FOOT AND ANKLE JOINT

Ankle joint is formed between distal articulating surfaces of tibia – fibula – proximal articulating surface of talus. Foot is divided into hindfoot (talus and calcaneum), midfoot (Navicular bone, cuboid and three cuneiform bones) and forefoot (five metatarsals and phalanges).

Fracture patterns of calcaneum and talus can be well demonstrated by CT scan. Tarsal coalition, osteochondral lesions and various plantar arch deformities are also well seen.

CT HIP JOINTS

NORMAL ANATOMY

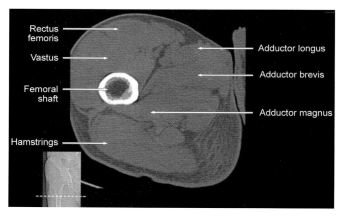

Figure 10.1: Axial CT section of hip

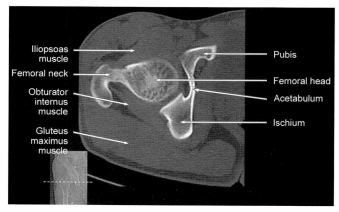

Figure 10.2: Axial CT section of hip

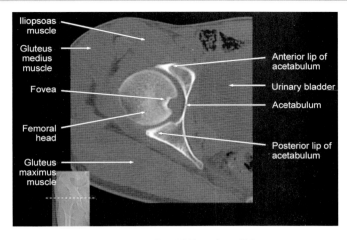

Figure 10.3: Axial CT section of hip

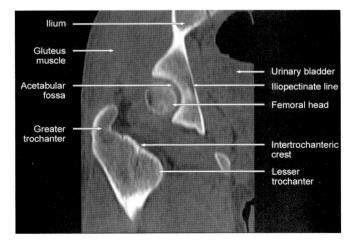

Figure 10.4: Coronal CT recon of hip

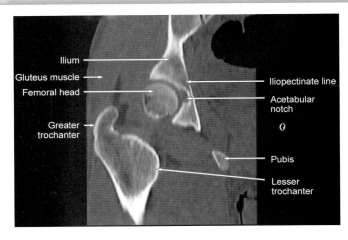

Figure 10.5: Coronal CT recon of hip

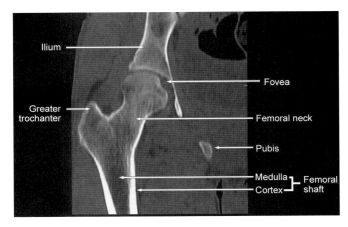

Figure 10.6: Coronal CT recon of hip

CT KNEE

NORMAL ANATOMY

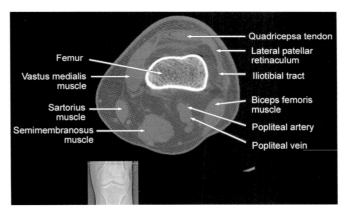

Figure 10.7: Axial CT section of knee

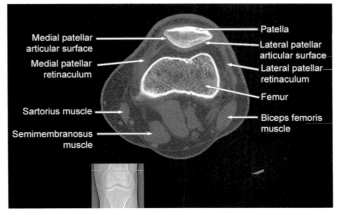

Figure 10.8: Axial CT section of knee

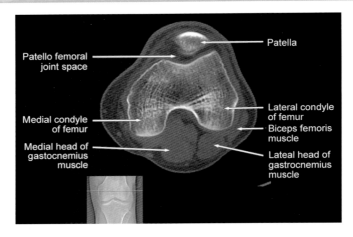

Figure 10.9: Axial CT section of knee

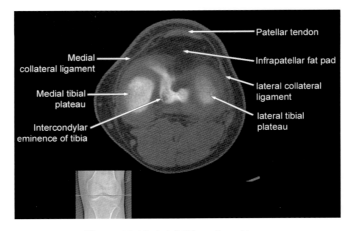

Figure 10.10: Axial CT section of knee

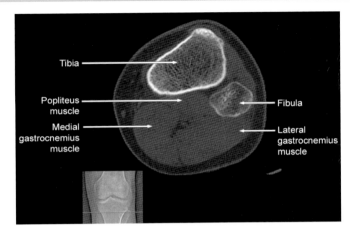

Figure 10.11: Axial CT section of knee

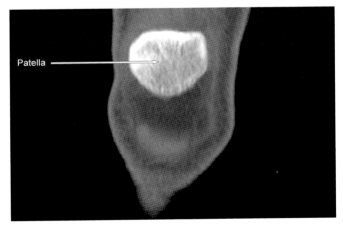

Figure 10.12: Coronal CT recon of knee

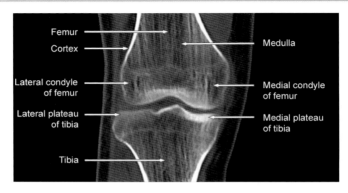

Figure 10.13: Coronal CT recon of knee

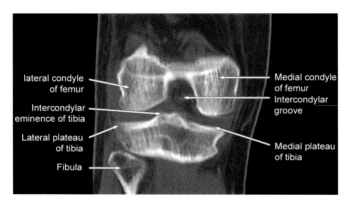

Figure 10.14: Coronal CT recon of knee

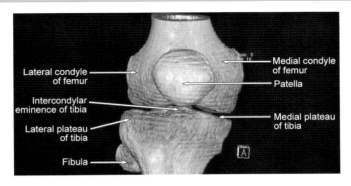

Figure 10.15: Volume rendered CT recon of knee
(Anteroposterior projection)

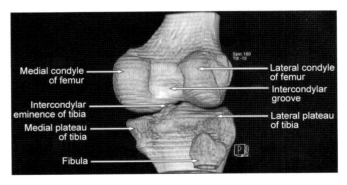

Figure 10.16: Volume rendered CT recon of knee
(Posteroanterior oblique projection)

CT FOOT AND ANKLE

NORMAL ANATOMY

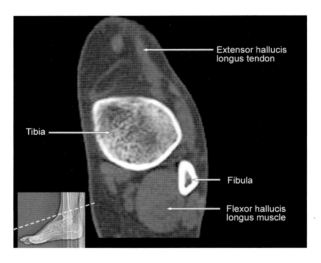

Figure 10.17: Axial CT section of foot

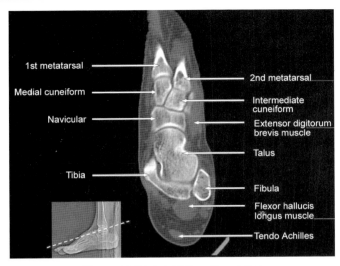

Figure 10.18: Axial CT section of foot

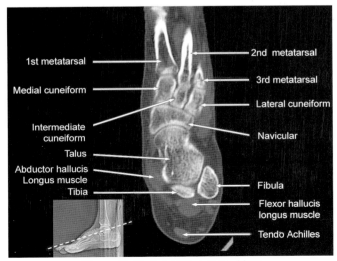

Figure 10.19: Axial CT section of foot

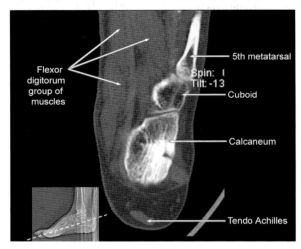

Figure 10.20: Axial CT section of foot

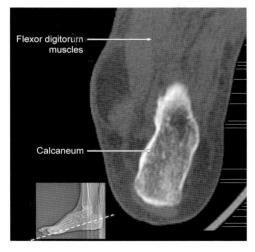

Figure 10.21: Axial CT section of foot

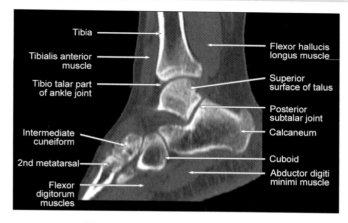

Figure 10.22: Sagittal CT recon of foot

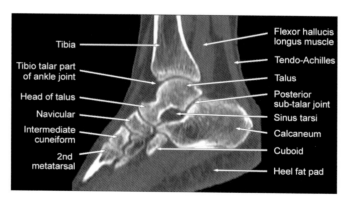

Figure 10.23: Sagittal CT recon of foot

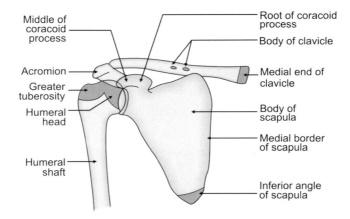

Middle of coracoid process

Acromion

Greater tuberosity

Humeral head

Humeral shaft

Root of coracoid process

Body of clavicle

Medial end of clavicle

Body of scapula

Medial border of scapula

Inferior angle of scapula

Figure 11.1: Shoulder joint

Shoulder Joint

BONES	OSSIFICATION	
Body of Scapula	8th Week of Fetal Life	
Body of Clavicle (two centers)	5th and 6th Week of Fetal Life	
Shaft of Humerus	8th Week of Fetal Life	

EPIPHYSIS	APPEARANCE	FUSION
Head of Humerus	1 year	
Greater Tuberosity	3 years	
Lesser Tuberosity	5 years	
Acromian Process	15-18 years	25th year
Middle of Coracoid Process	1 year	15th year
Root of Coracoid Process	17 years	25th year
Inferior Angle of Scapula	14-20 years	22-25 years
Medial Border of Scapula	14-20 years	22-25 years
Medial End of Clavicle	18-20 years	25th year

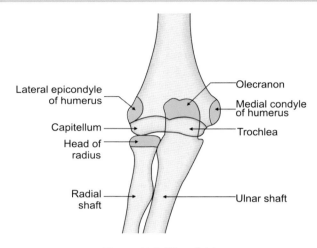

Figure 11.2: Elbow joint

Elbow Joint

BONES	OSSIFICATION	
Radial Shaft	8th week of Fetal Life	
Ulnar Shaft	8th week of Fetal Life	
EPIPHYSIS	**APPEARANCE**	**FUSION**
Lateral epicondyle	10-12 years	17-18 years
Medial epicondyle	05-08 years	17-18 years
Capitellum	01-03 years	17-18 years
Head of Radius	05-06 years	16-19 years
Trochlea	11th year	18th year
Olecranon process	10-13 years	16-20 years

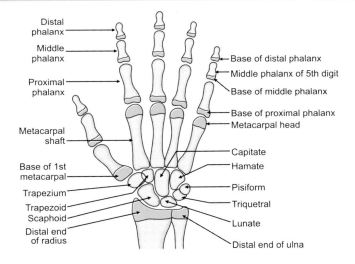

Figure 11.3: Wrist and hand

Wrist and Hand

BONES	OSSIFICATION	
Capitate	4 months	
Hamate	4 months	
Triquetral	3 years	
Lunate	4-5 years	
Trapezium	6 years	
Trapezoid	6 years	
Pisiform	11 years	
Metacarpals	10th Week of Fetal Life	
Proximal Phalanges	11th Week of Fetal Life	
Middle Phalanges	12th Week of Fetal Life	
Distal Phalanges	9th Week of Fetal Life	
Middle Phalanx of 5th Digit	14th Week of Fetal Life	

EPIPHYSIS	APPEARANCE	FUSION
Lower End of Radius	1-2 years	20th year
Lower End of Ulna	5-8 years	20th year
Metacarpal Heads	2.5 years	20th year
Base of Proximal Phalanges	2.5 years	20th year
Base of Middle Phalanges	3 years	18-20 years
Base of Distal Phalanges	3 years	18-20 years
Base of 1st Metacarpal	2.5 years	20th year

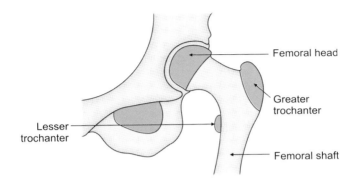

Figure 11.4: Hip joint

HIP Joint

BONES	OSSIFICATION	
Proximal Femoral Shaft	7th Week of Fetal Life	
EPIPHYSIS	**APPEARANCE**	**FUSION**
Femoral Head	1 year	18-20 years
Greater Trochanter	3-5 years	18-20 years
Lesser Trochanter	8-14 years	18-20 years

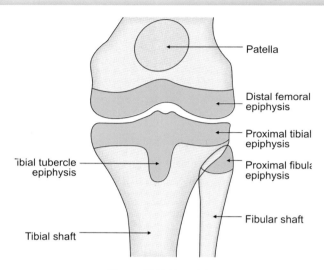

Figure 11.5: Knee joint

Knee Joint

BONES	OSSIFICATION	
Tibial Shaft	7th Week of Fetal Life	
Fibular Shaft	8th Week of Fetal Life	
Patella	5 years	

EPIPHYSIS	APPEARANCE	FUSION
Proximal Tibia	At Birth	20th year
Tibial Tubercle	5-10 years	20th year
Proximal Fibular	4th year	25th year
Distal Femoral	At Birth	20th year

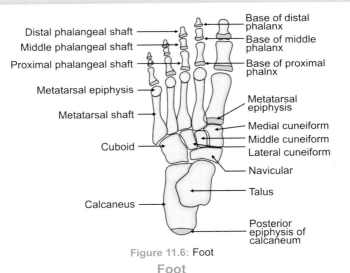

Figure 11.6: Foot

Foot

BONES	OSSIFICATION
Calcaneus	6th Month of Fetal Life
Talus	6th Month of Fetal Life
Navicular	3-4 years
Cuboid	At Birth
Lateral Cuneiform	1 year
Middle Cuneiform	3 years
Medial Cuneiform	3 years
Metatarsal Shafts	8th-9th week of Fetal Life
Phalangeal Shafts	10th week of Fetal Life

EPIPHYSIS	APPEARANCE	FUSION
Metatarsals	3 years	17-20 years
Proximal Phalangeal Base	3 years	17-20 years
Middle Phalangeal Base	3 years	17-20 years
Distal Phalangeal Base	5 years	17-20 years
Posterior Calcaneal	5 years	At Puberty

12 Radiation Exposure and Protection

As per the International System of units, dose of ionizing radiation is measured in unit called as gray (Gy). One Gy is defined as that quantity of radiation which results in energy deposition of one joule per kilogram in the irradiated tissue. Gray has replaced the earlier unit known as the rad. 1Gy is equal to 100 rad.

Effective dose of radiation is different for different tissues and is measured in terms of a unit called as Sieverts (Sv). This depends on the quality factor (Q) of the tissue which permits passage of energy.

$$\text{Dose equivalent (Sv)} = \text{Quality factor (Q)} \times \text{Dose (Gy)}$$

Average Effective Dose in mSv

- X-ray Chest - 0.02
- CT Orbits - 0.8
- CT Temporal bone - 1.0
- CT Head - 2.0
- CT Spine - 3.0
- CT Chest - 8.0
- CT Abdomen - 10.0
- CT Pelvis - 10.0

Effects of Radiation Exposure

- Deterministic effects are those which increase in severity with dose and include cataracts, blood dyscrasias and impaired fertility.

- Stochastic effects of radiation are the ones whose probability of effect rather than severity increases with dose and include cancer and genetic effects.
- However, since radiation exposure entails inherent risks of radiation effects, no decision to expose an individual can be undertaken without weighing benefits of exposure against potential risks, that is, making a benefit risk analysis.
- Ten Day Rule – All females of reproductive age who need an X-ray examination should get it done within first 10 days of menstrual cycle to avoid irradiation of possible conception.
- Radiography of area remote from fetus can be done safely at any time during pregnancy.
- Atomic Energy Regulatory Body (AERB) recommends that once a pregnancy is established the dose equivalent to surface of pregnant woman's abdomen should not exceed 2 mSv for the remainder of the pregnancy.

Principles of Radiation Protection

- Justification of a practice, e.g. the benefit to risk ratio is high for CT brain in cerebrovascular hemorrhage and low in screening mammography in women below 35 years.
- Optimized Protection "Optimization of the radiological procedure" is to reduce radiation exposures to the minimum levels. This optimization is possible by good quality assurance and quality control.
- Dose limitation by using high frequency generators which enable "high kV and low mAs technique.

The Triad of Radiation Protection Actions

Time – The exposure time is related to radiation exposure and exposure rate (exposure per unit time) as:

Exposure = Exposure rate × Time

Distance – Distance is between the source of radiation and the exposed individual. The exposure to the individual decrease inversely as the square of the distance. This is known as the inverse square law.

Shielding – Shielding implies that certain materials (concrete, lead) will attenuate radiation (reduce its intensity) when they are placed between the source of radiation and the exposed individual.

13 CT Contrast Media

I. IODINATED INTRAVASCULAR AGENTS

Intravascular radiological contrast media are iodine containing chemicals which add to the details from any given CT scan study and thereby aid in the diagnosis. They were first introduced by Moses Swick. Iodine (atomic weight 127) is an ideal choice element for X-ray absorption because the k shell binding energy of iodine (33.7) is nearest to the mean energy used in diagnostic radiography and thus maximum photoelectric interactions can be obtained which are a must for best image quality.

These compounds after intravascular injection are rapidly distributed by capillary permeability into extravascular extra-cellular space and almost 90 % is excreted by glomerular filtration by kidneys within 12 hours.

Following iodinated contrast media are available:

1. Ionic monomers, e.g. Diatrizoate, Iothamalate, Metrizoate.
2. Non-ionic monomers, e.g. Iohexol, Iopamidol, Iomeron.
3. Ionic dimer, e.g. Ioxaglate.
4. Non-ionic dimmer, e.g. Iodixanol, Iotrolan.

The amount of contrast required is usually 1-2 ml/kg body weight.

Normal osmolality of human serum is 290 mOsm/kg. Ionic contrast media have much higher osmolality than normal human serum and are known as High Osmolar Contrast Media (HOCM), while non-ionic contrast media have lower osmolality than

Atlas of Human Anatomy on CT Imaging

normal human serum and are known as Low Osmolar Contrast Media (LOCM).

Side effects or adverse reactions to contrast media are divided as:

1. Idiosyncratic anaphylactoid reactions
2. Non-idiosyncratic reactions like nephrotoxicity and cardio-toxicity.

Adverse reactions are more with HOCM than LOCM. So LOCM are preferred.

Delayed adverse reactions although very rare are, however, more common with LOCM and include Iodide mumps, Systemic Lupus Erythematosus (SLE) and Stevens-Johnson syndrome.

Principles of treatment of adverse reaction involves mainly five basic steps: ABCDE

A – Maintain proper airway
B – Breathing – Support for adequate breathing
C – Maintain adequate circulation. Obtain an IV access.
D – Use of appropriate drugs like antihistaminics for urticaria, atropine for vasovagal hypotension and bradycardia, beta agonists for bronchospasm, hydrocortisone etc.
E – Always have emergency back up ready including ICU care.

II. BARIUM SULPHATE

Barium sulphate suspensions are used for evaluating gastrointestinal tract. Barium (atomic weight 127) is an ideal choice element for X-ray absorption because the k shell binding energy of barium (37) is near to the mean energy used in diagnostic radiography and thus maximum photoelectric interactions can be obtained which are a must for best image quality. Moreover, barium sulphate is non-absorbable, non-toxic and can be prepared into a stable suspension.

For CT scan of abdomen, 1000-1500 ml of 1-5% w/vol barium sulphate suspension is used.

Severe adverse reactions are rare. Rarely mediastinal leakage can lead to fibrosing mediastinitis while peritoneal leakage can cause adhesive peritonitis.

III. CARBON DIOXIDE

Rarely carbon dioxide is used for infradiaphragmatic CT angiography in patients who are sensitive to iodinated contrast.

14   Artifacts

An artifact is an abnormal looking/appearing false finding in an image and is unrelated to the patient. It is thus a ghost appearance and in reality it does not exist.

Motion artifacts occur due to patient's motion. Metal implants/ornaments give rise to streak artifacts or beam hardening artifacts due to which adjacent structural details are obscured. Ring artifacts occur due to problems in detectors. When a partial volume is sampled or included in the field of view of imaging it gives rise to partial volume artifact.

A. Angulation artifact seen as the asymmetric appearance of frontal horns of lateral ventricles as head was not symmetrically positioned. In reality, both ventricles are equal in size and are symmetrical (Fig. 14.1).

B. Partial volume artifact seen as symmetric hyperdensities in the frontal region is due to partial volume of the bone (Fig. 14.2).

C. Ring artifacts occur as a result of detector malfunction which could either be due to improper calibration or due to detector-data ring mismatch. The center of the detector arc is the most sensitive region where ring artifacts can occur (Fig. 14.3).

D. Motion artifact due to accidental motion of right hand by patient (Fig. 14.4).

E. Streak artifacts due to metallic implant in tibia (Fig. 14.5).

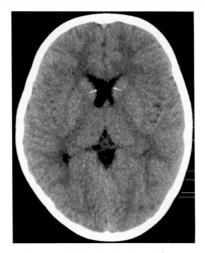

Figure 14.1: Angulation artifact

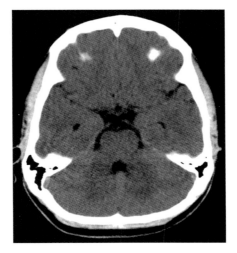

Figure 14.2: Partial volume artifact

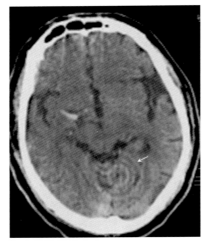

Figure 14.3: Ring artifact

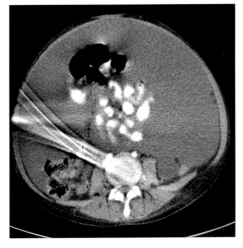

Figure 14.4: Motion artifact

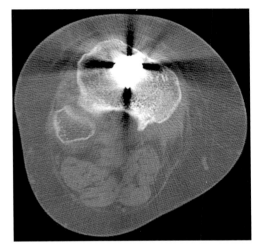

Figure 14.5: Streak artifact

INDEX